Images of Nurses

Perspectives from History, Art, and Literature

Images of Nurses

Perspectives from History, Art, and Literature

Edited by Anne Hudson Jones

uηη

University of Pennsylvania Press
Philadelphia

A complete listing of permissions to quote from copyrighted material (considered as part of the copyright page) can be found at the back of this volume.

Library of Congress Cataloging-in-Publication Data

Images of nurses.

"A Diebel memorial volume"—T.p. verso.
Includes index.
1. Nurses in art. 2. Nursing—Social aspects.
I. Jones, Anne Hudson. [DNLM: 1. History of Nursing.
WY 11.1 I31]
NX652.N87   1988   700   87-19240
ISBN 0-8122-8078-4
ISBN 0-8122-1254-1 (pbk.)

A Diebel Memorial Volume
in honor
of
William M. Crawford, M.D.

Acknowledgment is gratefully made to Mrs. Glenella Diebel, who established a fund in memory of her son, Donny Rae Diebel, M.D. (1945–1971), to support the publication program of the Institute for the Medical Humanities at the University of Texas Medical Branch at Galveston.

Contents

Illustrations

Preface

In 1980 at the University of Texas Medical Branch, I first taught a segment of an interdisciplinary humanities course for graduate nurses that I called "Images of Nurses in American Literature and Film." The interest and enthusiasm of those students, who did excellent work in the course, convinced me that nurses are eager to learn about this aspect of their profession. In preparing for that course, I also learned how little research in this area had been done by humanities scholars.

An important contribution to scholarship came from Leslie A. Fiedler. For the second volume of the new annual journal *Literature and Medicine,* which took as its theme "Images of Healers," Fiedler, a contributing editor, wrote a feature article titled "Images of the Nurse in Fiction and Popular Culture." His essay is reprinted here (it is the only article in this collection that has been previously published) because he was the first major literary critic to turn his attention to images of nurses.

To encourage further work, I sought and obtained support from the Institute for the Medical Humanities and the Sid W. Richardson Foundation for the research project that has culminated in this book. I asked historians, art historians, and literary scholars to write articles about images of nurses in their respective fields and then to come to Galveston to read and discuss each other's work. The result was even more exciting than I had hoped. Nurses and humanists—most of them feminist scholars—worked across disciplinary lines to establish a language free from jargon and to begin a dialogue that has enriched the subsequently revised essays that appear here. The working sessions in Galveston were, for me, like an ideal model of interdisciplinary women's studies scholarship come to life. The sessions could not have been such a success without the excellent work and energetic commitment of the participants. It has been a great personal and professional pleasure for me to work with them.

There are others whose help has been vital. Without the support of Ronald A. Carson, Director of the Institute for the Medical Humanities, this book would not have been possible. For their financial support, I am grateful to both the Sid W. Richardson Foundation, which provided the initial funding, and the Diebel Fund, which provided funding for the purchase of the many illustrations that accompany the text. For their help in typing various stages of the manuscript, I thank former Institute staff members Beverly Harvey and Jo Pope. For her help with proofreading, I thank Donna Polisar. For their very special help, in ways too numerous to elaborate, I thank Institute staff members Kathleen Stephens and Betty Herman. Finally, for her enthusiasm and excellent criticism, I thank Carol Gino; many essays in this book are the better for her comments and suggestions.

I hope that readers of this book will experience some of the same excitement of discovery that I have so enjoyed during my work on this project.

Contributors

Rima D. Apple, a Fellow in the Department of the History of Medicine and member of the Women's Studies Program of the University of Wisconsin—Madison, writes and lectures on a variety of topics in the history of medicine. She has published the *Illustrated Catalogue of the Slide Archive of Historical Medical Photographs at Stony Brook, Center for Photographic Images of Medicine and Health Care* (Westport, Conn.: Greenwood Press, 1984) and *Mothers and Medicine: A Social History of Infant Feeding, 1890–1950* (Madison: University of Wisconsin Press, 1987). She is working on a history of the commercial development of vitamins in the United States, 1920–1980s.

Joanne Trautmann Banks is Research Professor of Humanities at the University of Richmond. She also holds faculty appointments in the Departments of Medicine at the Medical College of Virginia and at the University of Virginia. Until 1986 she was Professor of Humanities and English at The Pennsylvania State University College of Medicine. For many years she has written widely about the relationships between literature and medicine. Her books in the field are *Literature and Medicine: An Annotated Bibliography* and *Healing Arts in Dialogue.* She is a founding editor of the journal *Literature and Medicine,* and editor of its fifth volume, *Use and Abuse of Literary Concepts in Medicine* (1986). Among her other work is the six-volume *Letters of Virginia Woolf,* of which she is co-editor.

Leslie A. Fiedler is Samuel Clemens Professor of English at the State University of New York at Buffalo. Among his many well-known works of fiction and literary criticism are *Love and Death in the American Novel* and *Freaks: Myths and Images of the Secret Self.* His two most recent books are *What Was Literature? Class Culture and Mass Society* and *Olaf Stapledon: A Man Divided.* He is also a contributing editor to the journal *Literature and Medicine.*

Darlene Clark Hine is John A. Hannah Professor of History at Michigan State University. Already the author of two books, she has recently received an ACLS Fellowship and a Fellowship from the National Humanities Center (1986–87) to complete her work on a book-length manuscript about the history of black women in the nursing profession. She is also the editor of *Black Women in the Nursing Profession: An Anthology of Historical Sources* (1984) and *The State of Afro-American History, Past, Present and Future* (1986).

Kathryn Montgomery Hunter is Associate Professor of Humanities in Medicine at the University of Rochester School of Medicine and Dentistry. Her research interests include satire in graphic art and the relation of the humanities to the study and practice of medicine. She has published articles in *Literature and Medicine, Shakespeare Quarterly, Studies in Eighteenth-Century Culture,* the *Journal of Medical Education,* and other scholarly journals. She is working on a study of the uses of narrative in medicine titled *The Patient as Text.*

Anne Hudson Jones is Associate Professor of Literature and Medicine at the Institute for the Medical Humanities of the University of Texas Medical Branch at Galveston. A founding editor of the journal *Literature and Medicine,* she edited its second volume, *Images of Healers* (1983); she is now the journal's General Editor. She has also published many articles on women writers and images of women in literature, as well as on various aspects of literature and medicine. She is completing two books, a reader's guide to the fiction of Kate Wilhelm and *Medicine and the Physician in American Popular Culture: A Reference Guide.*

Natalie Boymel Kampen is one of the organizers of the Women's Studies Program at the University of Rhode Island, where she is Professor of Art History and Women's Studies. She has published numerous articles on Roman sculpture and on women in art, as well as a book, *Image and Status,* about representations of Roman working women. With the aid of fellowships from the National Endowment for the Humanities and the Fulbright Commission, she is currently writing a book on historical subject matter in Roman provincial sculpture.

Karen Kingsley is Associate Professor of Architectural History in the School of Architecture, Tulane University. She has published articles on the iconography of women in art, and on medieval and modern architecture; she wrote the Design column for the *Times-Picayune States-Item* and regularly writes on architecture for other public-interest magazines. She is curator of two traveling exhibitions, one on architecture of the 1930s and the other on nineteenth-century Southern women.

Barbara Melosh is Associate Curator in the Division of Medical Sciences, National Museum of American History, Smithsonian Institution and Associate Professor of English and American Studies, George Mason

University. She is the author of *"The Physician's Hand": Work Culture and Conflict in American Nursing* (Temple University Press, 1982) and has compiled and introduced an anthology of nine stories with nurse characters, *American Nurses in Fiction* (Garland Press, 1984).

Janet Muff is a psychotherapist, practicing in southern California. Most of her clients are women and many are nurses. She lectures nationally on women's issues and consults with various organizations in the areas of psychiatric–mental health nursing practice and conflict management. Her book *Socialization, Sexism, and Stereotyping: Women's Issues in Nursing* (C. V. Mosby, 1982) received an *American Journal of Nursing* Book-of-the-Year Award in 1983.

Introduction

This book is divided into three parts. The first part deals with images of nurses in the visual arts; the second, with literary images of nurses; and the third, with the complex interactions between social issues, such as racism and sexism, and images of nurses. Together, these essays consider images from approximately twenty-five centuries, from the fifth century B.C. through the twentieth century. Yet despite the range and diversity of the essays, certain major themes come up repeatedly. The most basic is that nursing is the quintessential female profession, having its etymological and cultural origins in the biological aspects of femaleness. The first nurses were mothers. The second, as Natalie Boymel Kampen shows us in the art of ancient Greece and Rome, were wet nurses, or baby nurses, women who nursed other women's children. From this literal nourishing, the meaning of "to nurse" expanded, by metaphor, to include caring for the sick as well as for children. Nursing began in the home, a natural part of women's familial and domestic duties. No matter how highly technical and skilled modern nursing has become, the profession still carries with it the connotations of its name. As Leslie A. Fiedler points out, "not merely . . . does Nurse equal Woman, but, on an even profounder mythological level, Woman equals Nurse." As Kathryn Montgomery Hunter observes, female nurses as characters in literature are *always* symbolic, of Woman, writ large. And as Janet Muff says: "The issues that concern nurses are women's issues (and vice versa)."

Another important theme that recurs in the essays is that of nursing as female power, which both attracts and repels. Because nurses are associated with illness and death, they evoke fears of helplessness and mortality. In illness, patients often regress to a childlike state, thus reinforcing the image of nurse as mother and calling up the strong emotions and conflicts of the mother-child relationship. The nurse has power over patients whose illnesses make them dependent on her. When the nurse is female and the patient is male, the inverted sex roles, as Barbara Melosh calls them, can lead to erotic fantasies. When nurses are not imaged as mothers, then, they are often imaged as lovers.

The work of nursing is intimate, allowing nurses to violate usual social taboos by seeing and touching private parts of their patients' bodies. It was no accident that when *Playboy* magazine decided for the first time in its history to run a cover—for the November 1983 issue—using only a woman's face (and not her nearly nude body), the face was that of a nurse, so identified by her nurse's cap. This image of nurse as erotic sex object derives, in large part, from male fantasies based on nurses' occupational necessity of handling human (male) bodies. Yet the same bodily intimacy that produces erotic images of nurses can also lead nurses themselves, through their closeness to the mortality of other human beings, to a spiritual transcendence that represents nursing at its best. These conflicting images of nurses, however we label them, reflect the general cultural confusion about women, who have traditionally been dichotomized into stereotypes of angelic mothers or evil seductresses, the Madonna or the whore. Men may want angels at their bedsides, but they do not want them in their beds.

In England in the late nineteenth century, Florence Nightingale was fighting against the prevailing stereotype of the nurse as a drunken, promiscuous bawd. The only other image of nursing at the time was of nurse as nun. Nightingale tried to combine elements of the monastic and military traditions to create a secular image of the nurse that was respectable enough for young women of the middle (and even upper) classes to choose nursing as a profession without suffering social disgrace and opprobrium. She succeeded beyond all reasonable expectation, and the image of her own figure carrying the lamp at Scutari became the symbol of professional nursing that has reigned for almost a century. When contemporary nurses reject this image as an archaic stereotype, they are still hard pressed to find an image with which to replace it. Apart from Nightingale's lamp, only the nursing uniform, cap, and pin are widely recognized visual symbols of the profession.

Professional secular nursing began with Nightingale. To look at historical images of nurses in art and literature before then, we must look at images of women who nurse. Images of professional (registered) nurses do not appear in art and literature until this century. Even in twentieth-century works, it is sometimes difficult to make distinctions between registered and nonregistered nurses. The general public may not care about these distinctions, being content to consider as nurses all those who perform nursing duties, without differentiating among them according to education or degree. But most nurses *do* care, thus reflecting the concern with hierarchical distinctions that is a byproduct of contemporary nursing's attempt to elevate its professional status.

Many of the images of nurses discussed in these essays are negative ones. In this, they reflect general images of women. Yet nurses—even nursing leaders—have sometimes objected to studying negative images of nurses because such images are depressing. Not studying such images will not make them go away, however. To know and understand why the images are as they are is a first step toward both personal and professional self-knowledge for nurses. To know the past is to understand the present and to have hope for changing the future.

An important question then is what we can—or should—do about negative images of nurses. If we agree that only positive images of nurses should be presented (at least until we redress the balance somewhat), there are still problems. Whose positive image of the nurse should be presented? And for whom? We may not all agree on the ideal image of the nurse. Even if we did and if only ideal nurses were presented, what would happen when the public discovered that, in fact, real nurses are only human—not ideals? As an analogous example, physicians complained about Marcus Welby because patients who had seen Dr. Welby in action on television were often highly dissatisfied with their own physician's behavior toward them.

Also important, we risk reducing art to propaganda if we insist on certifying only certain kinds of images. The difference between image and stereotype may be an important guideline here. We do need to protest unthoughtful, clichéd stereotypes that prevent nurses from being recognized and appreciated as persons and as professionals. But we must be thoughtful about what we do lest we silence those (and nurses among them) whose stories we need to hear. The point is that nurses deserve respect as persons, not disregard as a preconceived type or class.

More than any other professional woman, the nurse is a metaphor for all women. The tensions within the profession of nursing today and the conflicting images of nurses reflect historical and contemporary conflicts about women's role. The many paired, opposing concepts and images that emerge in these essays—intimacy and eroticism, Madonna and whore, angel and bawd, spirituality and earthiness—are pertinent to an understanding of general women's history as well as to the history of nursing.

Thus, the final question: Can we expect to create images of nurses—still largely a gender-specific profession—that avoid the negativity associated with women's work? Probably not. The real solution to negative images of nurses must come from elevating the status of women and of all female labor. The issue, as Kathryn Montgomery Hunter raises it, is the social value of care—child care, care for the sick, care for the elderly, and care for the dying. Until such care, still associated almost exclusively with women and women's work, is properly valued in our society, nursing will not be either. The status of nursing, the status of women's work, and the status of women have been and will remain mutually dependent.

Images of Nurses

Perspectives from History, Art, and Literature

The three essays in Part I are devoted to images of nurses and nursing in the visual arts—in painting and sculpture, in photographs, and in architecture. The essays are arranged chronologically: the first begins with images in painting and sculpture from as long ago as the fifth century B.C. and ends with images from the seventeenth century; the second focuses on photographic images from the late nineteenth and early twentieth centuries; and the third traces the influence of late-nineteenth-century ideas about nursing on the twentieth-century architecture of nursing. Together these three essays provide a historical overview of images of nurses and nursing in the visual arts from ancient to contemporary times.

In each of the essays, the author introduces background concepts necessary to the study of the particular art form she considers. The most basic concept each author discusses is the relationship between the images of nurses in the visual arts and the historical and social reality of nurses and nursing. This relationship is not simple, nor is it the same for each of the art forms considered in this section.

Natalie Boymel Kampen's essay, "Before Florence Nightingale: A Prehistory of Nursing in Painting and Sculpture," opens Part I by examining the images of nurses in early painting, prints, and sculpture to see what they can explain about contemporary images of nurses and problems of nursing. The first art historian to study systematically these early images of women as health care workers, Kampen focuses on three phases in European art that are critical to an understanding of the image of the nurse: Greek and Roman antiquity from the fifth century B.C. to the fourth century A.D.; the Christian Middle Ages and Renaissance, fourteenth through sixteenth centuries; and seventeenth-century Flemish (Belgium).

Kampen points out that paintings and sculptures are not illustrations of the real world. Rather, images in paintings and sculptures have been refracted through the lens of the artist's eye. The artist conveys an image or concept that is uniquely his or hers, yet an image that is influenced by the social conditioning and artistic conventions of the place and time in which the artist lives. In the art of Greek and Roman antiquity, for example, the scenes that are usually depicted are of public events that women

3

did not attend. Thus, the nurse, when she appears at all in such art, is, as Kampen says so eloquently, a nameless conventional figure used to advance a narrative not her own. Even though art does not simply illustrate life, perhaps *because* it does not, its highly selective and carefully constructed images become a kind of visual shorthand that transmits our culture's commonly accepted notions and values from one generation to the next. Iconography, which Kampen defines as "the study of images as symbols or signs of ideas," can help us understand the significance of a given image or set of images.

In the next essay, "Image or Reality? Photographs in the History of Nursing," Rima D. Apple uses photographs as primary source documents for a historical analysis of American nursing. Because women's lives have not always been part of the record of public events the way men's lives have been, women's scholarship has had to devise new methods to deal with unconventional sources, such as these photographs, to give us insight into women's—and thus nurses'—daily lives. Apple focuses on the image of hospital nurses in the late nineteenth and early twentieth centuries and finds that the photographic evidence shows a daily life of nurses that is not conveyed by written sources. In some cases photographs reinforce stereotypes of the time, but in other cases they lead us to question the usually accepted interpretations of the history of nursing.

The relationship between photographic images and reality is different from the relationship between painting and sculpture and reality. Apple points out that photographs are considered more realistic than paintings because they are more objective. Yet even though the camera never lies, or so we are told, the photographer exerts more control over the image his or her camera produces than might at first be evident. Posed arrangements of people and places may present an idealized image far different from the everyday reality. But just as the lies people choose to tell can reveal much about them, the photographic images nurses and photographers choose to present are intriguing—whether an image is an exact representation of reality or not. All this notwithstanding, unposed, candid photographs offer the nearest thing to a realisitic image we can get. For unposed, candid images the important questions are what was photographed (and by implication, what was not)—and why.

Part I closes with Karen Kingsley's essay, "The Architecture of Nursing." Kingsley is the first architecture historian to attempt a synthetic study of the origins and developments of the nurses' residence and school as an architectural type in the late nineteenth and then the twentieth centuries. She finds that many of the important issues in the history of professional nursing are reflected in these architectural designs. Architecture has been used to keep nurses in their place, both literally and figuratively.

The relationship between the architecture of nursing and the reality of nursing is even more complex than the relationships between images of nurses in painting and sculpture and reality, or between photographic images of nurses and reality. As Kingsley explains, architecture serves as a visual symbol that reflects the importance of an activity or an institution within its culture. The exterior of a building and its ornamental features can inspire the public's respect. The way the interior space of a building is organized controls the physical reality of its occupants and influences their social interactions. A building of its own was important to the development of nursing as a profession not just to house and protect nurses, but also to stand as a visual representation of nurses and their profession to the general public.

Natalie Boymel Kampen

1. Before Florence Nightingale: A Prehistory of Nursing in Painting and Sculpture*

The nurse is a woman all in white with a small cap on her head; she looks out from book covers, cartoon frames, and television screens in the same costume—a visual stereotype most Americans think of as eternal. But the nurse's image was not always this antiseptic white one. In Western art, nurses have a complicated history, invisible in many periods, hard to recognize in others, and only in this century assuming the look we take for granted. To my knowledge, no art historian has studied the early image of the nurse in paintings, prints, and sculpture (in high art, that is) until now, and certainly no one has examined the images to see what they can explain about the history of nursing and the present situation, status, and representation of nurses.[1]

My focus in this essay is on the history of art that represents women as health care workers in the time before Florence Nightingale. Rather than presenting a survey of images from all periods, I have chosen to focus on three phases in European art: Greek and Roman from the fifth century B.C. to the fourth century A.D.; the late Medieval and Renaissance (especially the fifteenth and sixteenth centuries); and the seventeenth-century Flemish (modern Belgium). As I will show, these three periods are not necessarily representative of all art history, but they are critical to an understanding of how the image of the nurse came into being. Antiquity had

*I wish to thank the following people for their help in the preparation of this essay: Jules Boymel, John Dunnigan, Carol Gino, and Elizabeth Grossman all read it at various stages and made invaluable comments; Karin Abatecola Messier, acting as research assistant, found important material and saved me many hours of work; and directors of many museums and research institutes provided photographs and data as cited in the captions and footnotes.

no pictures of women who cared for the sick; these evolved much later, in the Christian Middle Ages and Renaissance, and they were due to the existence of new conditions in religion, society, and art more than to changes in nursing itself. The new Christian nursing picture preserved ideas from earlier periods and helped to carry into our own time some important stereotypes: nursing as woman's natural work, as domestic work, as a selfless act of love and devotion. To understand these early images is to see more clearly some of the sources of nursing's current identity crisis.

The picture in the mind's eye, of that woman in white or of Florence Nightingale in her billowing dark cloak, is not the same as the reality of nursing now or a hundred years ago. The way of investigating pictures of nurses in the history of art makes that distinction—between art and reality—very emphatically. Iconography, the study of images as symbols or signs of ideas, is based on the premise that a picture reflects the real world through a series of lenses. The artist's eye, her or his beliefs and social conditioning, her or his artistic heritage, and the conventions and unconscious patterns of representing standard forms all transform reality into the special and separate thing that is the artistic image. This study will look at the pictures not as illustrations of the real world but as metaphors, analogues, and parallel worlds in which reality is creatively reinterpreted. We will not see things that really existed unless artists and their patrons wanted to see those things, and when we see them, they will often be reshaped so that they refuse to answer our contemporary questions. This essay will suggest some of the questions the images *can* answer and some ways to ask those questions. It will, I hope, suggest directions for further investigations into the art history of nursing.

The Greek and Roman Tradition

Nursing the sick was never seen as a professional activity by people in the ancient world. Greek and Roman doctors—usually male—attended serious or complicated cases; midwives—always female—attended births and newborns; and female kin cared for the sick in the context of the family and without pay.[2] What this meant for the visual arts was that doctors and midwives were shown, but family members were not. A major reason for

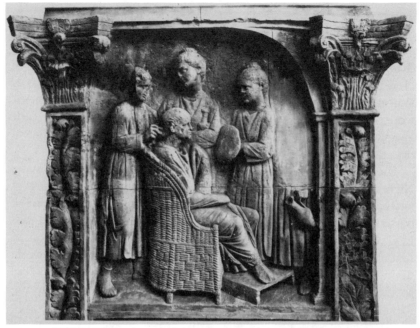

FIGURE 1-1. Roman Funerary Pillar, detail of woman with servants. Third century A.D. Trier, Rheinisches Landesmuseum. Photo F.U. 11016 F, courtesy Fototeca Unione, at the American Academy in Rome.

the absence of these kinswomen is artistic convention, the traditional ways of seeing and representing, which were passed down from one generation of artists to the next until they became unquestioned habits. For the most part, ancient artists gave form to public actions and events; they showed the world of men and of gods. In the rare cases when they painted and sculpted domestic scenes, they generally chose serene and pleasant moments. Greek vases of the later fifth century B.C. show women dressing, talking, and playing with children; Roman artists give us dinners at home and women having their hair done (Fig. 1-1).[3] We are never permitted to see the sick slaves being nursed by women in the villa infirmaries described by Roman writers; nowhere do we find any illustration of the passages in Roman historians that tell of women nursing men wounded in battle.[4] (The only exception to the rule, and it is an important one, is the scene of women mourning the dead and preparing their bodies for burial; the theme appears in Greek and Roman art as testimony to the public importance of this female role.) The conventions of classical art thus prevented both respectable women and their domestic slaves from being seen performing most unpleasant or onerous tasks, even though written evidence tells us that such activities were a normal part of women's household duties.

Only two kinds of scenes show women caring for the health of others in ancient art: childbirth and the infant's bath. In the childbirth scene, rare in Greek and Roman art, the patient is restrained by an assistant as the midwife works sitting or kneeling in front. In a small relief of the second century A.D. from a tomb at the Roman city of Ostia, near Rome, the patient sits on a birthing chair with handgrips while the midwife sits on a stool (Fig. 1-2); a statuette from sixth-century B.C. Cyprus puts the patient on the assistant's lap and shows the midwife kneeling before them (Fig. 1-3).[5] The scene of the infant's bath is far more common than the childbirth, especially in Roman art; a Roman second-century A.D. marble sarcophagus shows a typical scene, in which a woman bathes or lifts a newborn baby while his mother sits quietly looking on (Fig. 1-4).[6] The women who perform each of these jobs have different poses, actions, even costumes, and the two scene types are never shown on the same piece of sculpture.

Greek and Roman viewers looking at childbirth and bath scenes would have brought with them enough information to understand how different the two types were. Not only did the visual specifics differ (for example, midwives never wear the off-the-shoulder dress that is often seen on baby nurses), but the ideas the scenes projected were dissimilar as well. The childbirth could be either a mythological scene or one showing daily life, and the ancient viewer would know that the midwife was someone with skill and status. That information was part of the viewer's normal equipment; we know this from ancient medical writers and from inscriptions on tombstones set up for midwives. Soranus, the second-century A.D. writer on gynecology, discussed midwives as skilled and respected practitioners, while epitaphs praised them as honorable, competent members of the community.[7]

By contrast, baby nurses were usually slaves, servants who could be much loved in the family they worked for, but who were seldom, if ever, seen by society as independent professionals. They were nannies, and the scene of the baby's bath reflects their low status by subordinating and depersonalizing them. They become nameless conventional figures drawn from ancient mythology and theater rather than real life, and they are

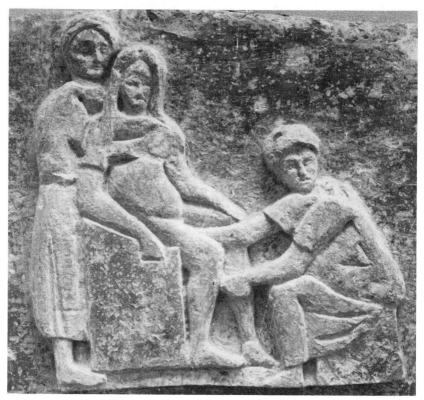

FIGURE 1-2. Roman Relief of a Childbirth Scene. Second century A.D. Ostia, Museo Ostiense. Photo F.U. 2388, courtesy Fototeca Unione, at the American Academy in Rome.

used, in art as in literature, to advance a narrative not their own.[8] The scene may be the bath of the infant wine god Dionysus, of the baby Alexander the Great, or of a wealthy Roman official in his first hours of life. It is just one of a series of standardized events, which show a hero's biography and his virtuous character. The baby nurse merely signals that we are seeing the infancy of a hero; she herself is no more individualized than the furniture—a subordinate in art and in reality.[9]

Art is mirroring some elements of reality here but not others. The different social status of midwives and baby nurses seems to influence their artistic forms and roles. In reality, however, and this comes again from Greek and Roman epitaphs and medical writers, midwives often did more than deliver babies. They could bathe and swaddle infants, care for moth-

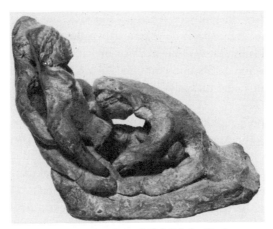

FIGURE 1-3. Greek Terracotta Figurine of Childbirth. Sixth century B.C. Nicosia, Cyprus Museum. Photo courtesy the Director of Antiquities and the Cyprus Museum.

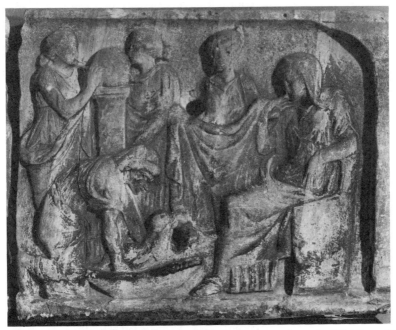

FIGURE 1-4. Roman *Biographical Sarcophagus,* with scenes from the life of an official, detail of the infant's bath. Late second century A.D. (ca. 180–90). Los Angeles County Museum of Art. Photo courtesy Los Angeles County Museum of Art, William Randolph Hearst Collection.

ers, and attend to all kinds of women's illnesses, but the visual images never reflect this.[10] By the same token, baby nurses could be replaced in many households by slaves-of-all-work or by female relatives; the art does not make these fine distinctions though. All we have are the two artistic types—baby nurse and midwife—and the subtleties of reality are lost beneath their surface.

The two iconographic elements, midwife and baby nurse, lived on through the Middle Ages and even into the seventeenth century. The midwife image was kept alive in illustrated health and medical texts as a standard teaching scene. In the thirteenth century, medical manuscripts were showing childbirth in exactly the same form it had had in antiquity. An illustration in an herbarium of the writer called Pseudo-Apuleius, now in the Austrian National Library in Vienna, shifts to a frontal view instead of the earlier profile but preserves all the other elements intact (Fig. 1-5).[11] The prints, both woodcuts and engravings, that illustrate fifteenth- and sixteenth-century books of instruction for midwives, such as Jacobus Rueff's *Trostbuechle* of 1554, continue to be based on the same artistic models and the same social attitude toward the midwife as a trained professional (Fig. 1-6).[12] Like her classical ancestors, she works outside her own family (a very unusual, even scandalous thing for women in the Middle Ages and Renaissance) but remains generally respectable because of her involvement with women and children.

The imagery of the baby nurse can also be traced without interruption from Roman tomb monuments of the second and third centuries to the sixteenth century. In every case, the baby nurse is shown in a domestic setting, and her depiction as a servant, kinswoman, or friend keeps her from taking on any special signs of professionalism. Early Christian and Byzantine art, from the fourth century to the fifteenth, took over the motif of the nurse bathing the baby for the Nativity of Christ, as in the eighth-century Byzantine ivory plaque now in the British Museum; drawing on the heroic images of the bath of the infant Alexander the Great as well as on Roman sarcophagi, Christian artists found an instantly recognizable way to communicate the epiphany of a new God-hero (Fig. 1-7).[13] The bath became a sign of Christ's special nature just as it had done for gods and heroes in antiquity.

Although the nurses in the Nativity of Christ fell into disuse in western Europe during the later Middle Ages, they continued to work in scenes of the Birth of the Virgin Mary and of John the Baptist. Encouraged by the

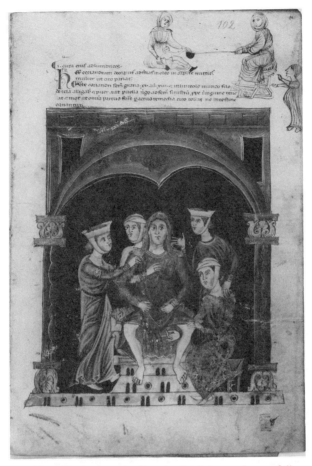

FIGURE 1-5. Medieval Herbarium, by Pseudo-Apuleius: codex 93, folio 102 recto, childbirth scene. Thirteenth century. Vienna, Austrian National Library. Photo courtesy Bild-Archiv und Porträt-Sammlung der Österreichische National-bibliothek, Vienna.

spread of the French cult of Mary with its special love for her and its inventions of new stories about her life, the representation of the Birth of the Virgin flourished all over Europe. In Italian versions of the fourteenth and fifteenth centuries, the event was shown taking place in an upper-class household populated with female attendants and visitors who came to congratulate the exhausted Saint Anne as she lay in bed. Andrea Orcagna's mid-fourteenth-century sculptural representation from Florence showed

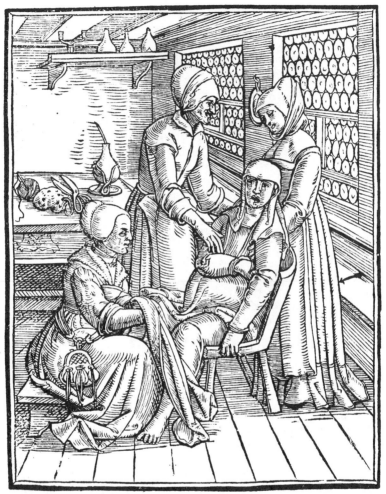

FIGURE 1-6. Renaissance Print of a Childbirth from Jacobus Rueff, *Ein schoen lustig Trostbuechle* (Zurich: C. Froschauer, 1554), folio 664 verso. Photo courtesy Wellcome Institute Library, London.

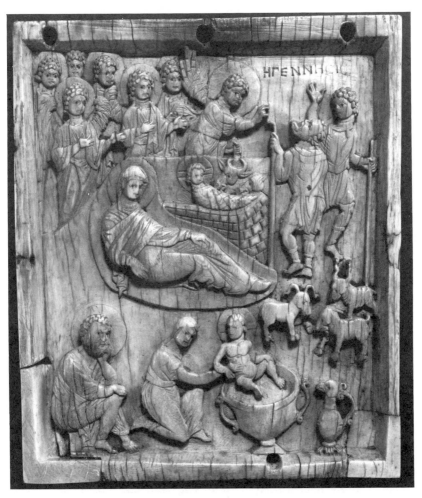

FIGURE 1-7. Byzantine Ivory Plaque with Nativity Scenes. Eighth century. London, British Museum. Photo courtesy Trustees of the British Museum.

the infant's bath in the foreground, where it would remain part of the scene throughout the Renaissance (Fig. 1-8).[14] Around the same time, the Birth of John the Baptist joined the Birth of the Virgin Mary as a favored scene. An illustrated prayer book by the fifteenth-century French painter Jehan Fouquet, the *Hours of Étienne Chevalier,* demonstrates the form and wide spread of the image with its elaborate domestic interiors and nurses always in attendance (Fig. 1-9).[15] Even into the next century, as in a German painting of the Birth of the Virgin by Albrecht Altdorfer, the nurse-maids bathing or caring for the baby continued to appear as household signs of the hero-god. Their status in these images is always subordinate, and no indications of professionalism ever remove them from the ranks of servants or relatives of low standing.

This first and longest chapter in the history of nurse imagery gives us no modern-style nurses at all. From ancient Greece until the fourteenth century, the only female health care workers in art were the midwives and baby nurses. None of the complicated realities of who did what, of women tending the wounded or the sick, of changing customs and skills, emerges in the works of art from this long moment. Only the shift from pagan myths and scenes of daily life to scenes of Christian subjects distinguishes early from late.

Late Medieval and Renaissance Art, Fourteenth through Sixteenth Centuries

As I have just shown, women of all classes who nursed the sick among their kin and dependents really had no distinctive visual iconography in antiquity or most of the Middle Ages. In the illustrated histories and health manuals or the popular prints of the later Middle Ages, women appeared with the sick to bring them their medicine or meals and to feed them (as in the fifteenth-century print *The Impatience of the Sick Man*) and watch over or pray for them while male physicians attended (as in the print by the Venetian artist Gentile Bellini *Visit to a Plague Victim,* 1493) (Fig. 1-10). No signs made clear which of the women were relatives as opposed to servants or hired nurses; the artistic and social legacy of the ancient world failed to provide later artists with any of the prototypes they needed to construct a recognizable iconography of domestic or professional sick care.[16]

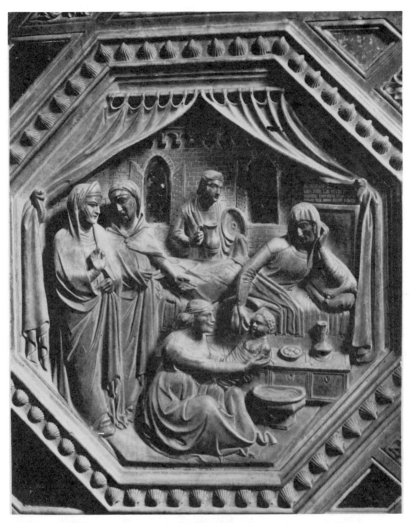

FIGURE 1-8. Andrea Orcagna, *Birth of the Virgin,* detail of Tabernacle. Fourteenth century. Florence, Church of Or S. Michele. Photo P.I.N. 2336, courtesy Alinari/Art Resource, New York.

It was only in the fourteenth and fifteenth centuries that a new, deeply Christian type of image for women as givers of health care came into being in Europe. As I will explain, changes in social, religious, and artistic ideas made possible the emergence of three themes: the Seven Corporal Works of Mercy, Saint Elizabeth nursing the sick, and the nursing sisters from

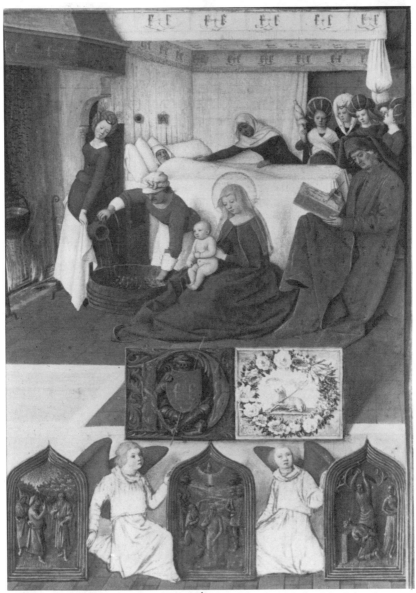

FIGURE 1-9. Jehan Fouquet, *Hours of Étienne Chevalier,* Birth of St. John the Baptist: manuscript 71 folio 7. Fifteenth century. Chantilly, Musée Condé. Photo RL 26751, courtesy Giraudon/Art Resource, New York.

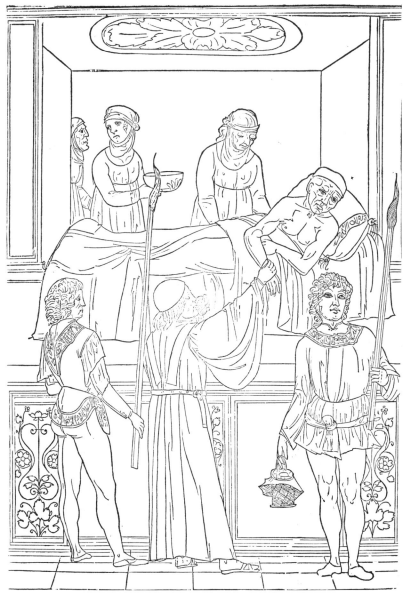

FIGURE 1-10. Gentile Bellini, *Visit to a Plague Victim*. 1493. Philadelphia Museum of Art. Photo courtesy Philadelphia Museum of Art, SmithKline Corporation Collection.

Christian hospitals. In considering each of these themes, I will show that the new nursing type employed visual elements that separated the nurse from her character as a family member or servant while still attaching her firmly to activities that were traditionally female and domestic. In other words, the nurse still attended to food, laundry, baths, bandages, and spiritual comfort, just as kinswomen did and still do; she served—but outside her own family and in ways that raised her religious or social standing. Her actions now found themselves in a new context and with new features rooted in an emphatically Christian theological iconography.

The Seven Corporal Works of Mercy appear in Christian writings from the twelfth century on; they were the acts that a Christian was to perform to bring bodily comfort to her or his fellow humans. Clothing the naked, feeding the hungry, housing the homeless, and visiting the sick were among these works of mercy that would help the Catholic win a place in heaven at the Day of Judgment.[17] The theme became popular in fifteenth- and sixteenth-century art in western Germany and the Netherlands because of its association with the Last Judgment; in this age of turbulence, when people feared the end of the world was near and when social rebellion and religious reform were spreading through northern Europe, the separation of the Blessed from the Damned was often on the lips of preachers and the minds of their flocks. Often shown as part of large-scale Last Judgment paintings, both in churches and town halls, the works of mercy carried with them hope for salvation in heaven and a sense of civic responsibility here on earth.[18] They had, as well, an attraction for artists, who were increasingly delighted by the look of the real world and real people; religion could be made part of everyday life in the pictures of the Seven Works.

All the concerns I have just noted are reflected in an important example by the anonymous Netherlandish painter, the Master of Alkmaar (Figs. 1-11, 1-12). His Last Judgment with *The Seven Works of Mercy,* painted in 1504, stresses the concreteness of good works performed by real people in the real world.[19] His scene "Visiting the Sick" gives an important depiction of women attending sick men who are neither their kin nor their masters. Here, finally, we are coming to a clear and direct nursing iconography. In the background, a man and a woman tend a naked invalid in a hospital ward with several beds. In the foreground, the second woman's outdoor cloak, her prosperous clothing, and her pose as she brings a cup into the ward all reinforce the distinction between caring for the sick as a family duty and as a Christian duty to those outside the family. The pop-

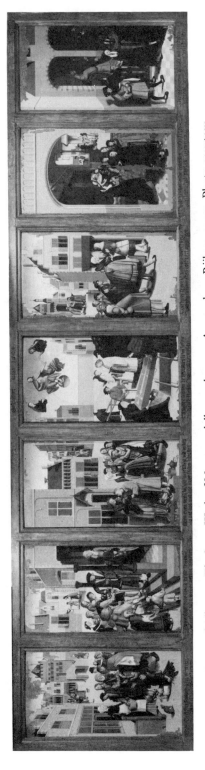

FIGURE 1-11. Master of Alkmaar, *The Seven Works of Mercy*, predella panels. 1504. Amsterdam, Rijksmuseum. Photo courtesy Rijksmuseum-Stichting.

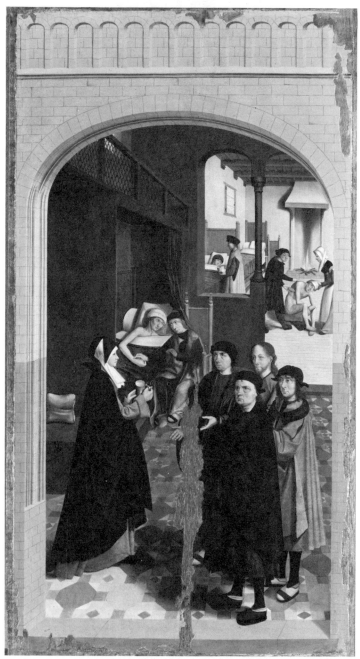

FIGURE 1-12. Master of Alkmaar, *The Seven Works of Mercy,* predella panel, "Visiting the Sick." 1504. Amsterdam, Rijksmuseum. Photo courtesy Rijksmuseum-Stichting.

ularity of the Seven Works of Mercy is especially significant in a time when city life and its contact with strangers increased and the needy were no longer always cared for by their kin. Pictures of the Seven Works by other artists follow the visual pattern seen in the Alkmaar Master's work, whether real men and women are represented or only anonymous types. What all the images show is the newly acceptable notion of a respectable woman visiting a sick neighbor, tending a sick stranger, doing her Christian duty in a public way.[20]

Saint Elizabeth visiting or caring for the sick represents a second late medieval and Renaissance contribution to the iconography of nursing. Although pictures of healing saints were very popular in the fifteenth and sixteenth centuries, only Elizabeth seems to have provided artists with a saintly model of a woman nursing as opposed to healing by laying on of hands, by surgery, or by miraculous intervention. By contrast with other healers, Saint Elizabeth normally appears performing some of the Seven Works of Mercy.[21] She gives her jewels to the poor as alms, gives bread to the hungry, and visits or nurses the sick. In this last case, the form is exactly the same as the motif in the Seven Works except that Elizabeth's halo identifies her as a saint. In a late fourteenth-century painting by an anonymous artist from the Rhineland, the saint feeds a sick man whose frail arms and chest are left bare by the bedclothes; feeding the hungry and nursing the sick combine two elements of the Works of Mercy and associate them with a famous and beloved saint to further dignify the iconography and the actions (Fig. 1-13).[22]

The third Christian nursing theme is the least obviously theological in character. The scenes of hospice and hospital sisters working in their wards combine elements of the Seven Works of Mercy and Saint Elizabeth with an interest in the appearance and experience of the hospital environment. With their love of details drawn from the seen world, they demonstrate the taste for the everyday and for accurate depiction of things and places that was typical of fifteenth-century northern European artists and patrons. It was this taste that made northern art so different both from the more traditional and less realistic art of the Middle Ages and from the more idealized art of the Italian Renaissance.

Several features common to scenes of nursing sisters help to define the nature of their role: they nurse patients who are most often men lying in bed; they work in a distinctive location that does not look like a house; they wear distinctive costumes; their activities are domestic and religious rather than specifically medical; and, most important, they are never subordinated to patients or doctors.

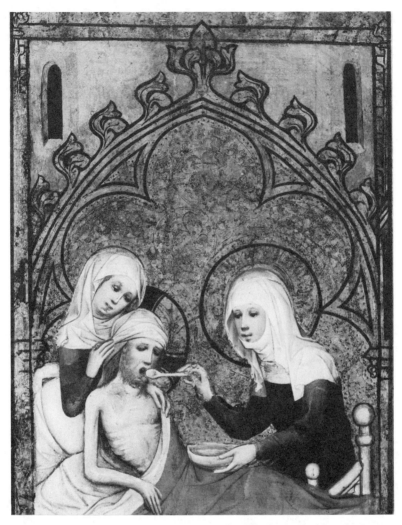

FIGURE 1-13. Anonymous Rhenish Painter, Saint Elizabeth Clothing the Poor and Caring for the Sick, detail of Caring for the Sick. Fourteenth century. Cologne, Wallraf-Richartz-Museums. Photo courtesy Rheinische Bildarchiv, Cologne.

An early appearance of the motif of the nursing sisters, which shows typical actions and setting, occurs in a mid-fourteenth-century drawing from Saint John's Hospital in the Belgian town of Bruges (Fig. 1-14).[23] There, two nursing sisters attend two male patients who lie in their beds; the one on the right is offering a bowl to her patient. The patient in bed

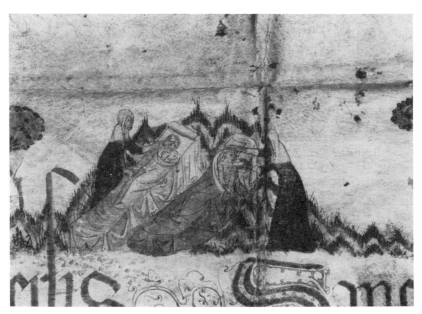

FIGURE 1-14. Drawing showing Nursing Sisters, detail 5. 1354. Bruges, Museum Onze-Lieve-Vrouw ter Potterie. Photo courtesy Openbaar Centrum voor Maatschapplijk Welzijn, Bruges.

identifies a nursing scene also in a page from a Parisian manuscript of about 1482 (Fig. 1-15). The manuscript, by Jehan Henry, offers spiritual counsel to the Augustinian nuns who nursed at the Hôtel-Dieu, the great general hospital in Paris. Among the pages showing the various vows of the sisters is one where groups of nuns stand with figures who represent four Virtues; they all gather before the beds of the sick in a ward.[24] Although no nursing takes place, the recognizable costumes with their white gowns and black veils, the beds with patients, and the emphasis on spiritual rather than purely physical treatment identify the scene as one of Christian hospital nursing.

Around 1500 an anonymous print from a church document of the Archbishop of Bourges in France presented a fully developed Christian ward scene. The Paris Hôtel-Dieu ward was shown as a large room with the sick in their beds in almost every corner; the sisters work among their patients, giving them food and drink, offering them prayers, and even sewing them into their shrouds (Fig. 1-16). Although the priest is present, there are no male physicians, nor is there evidence of anyone giving orders to the sis-

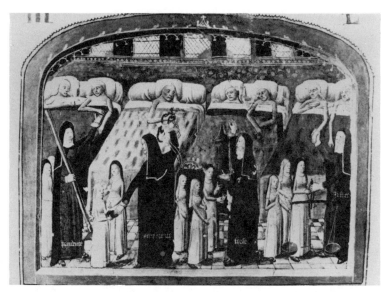

FIGURE 1-15. Jehan Henry, *Livre de la vie active des religieuses de l'Hôtel-Dieu de Paris,* Hospital Ward. Ca. 1482. Paris, Musée de l'Assistance Publique. Photo courtesy Cliché Assistance Publique.

ters. The Augustinians perform acts of mercy just as Saint Elizabeth did, their clothing and the location clear and easily identified. The experience of the hospital, with its emphasis on spiritual as well as physical care, combines with the iconography of the Seven Works of Mercy and the nursing saints for a new and distinctive image of the female nurse.

In Italy, despite strong contacts with northern Europe and its artists in the fifteenth century, the themes I have been discussing are rarely shown. Medicine apparently belonged to men and birthing and nursing to women, public to men and private to women. Evidence to that effect comes from an illustration in a fifteenth-century medical book from Ferrara, which shows a ward with three patients in beds, one ambulatory and one sitting up to be treated.[25] All the people caring for the sick are men, from the elegantly dressed physicians to the servant with a cup. The Seven Works of Mercy and female nursing saints are almost never shown in Italian Renaissance art, and female nurses, when shown at all, stand in the background and, as in Gentile Bellini's print with doctors visiting a plague victim, let the male doctors have the foreground (Fig. 1-10). Only one picture, Pontormo's wall painting for the Hospital of Saint Matthew in

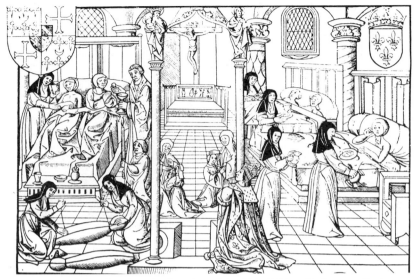

FIGURE 1-16. Print showing the Interior of the Hôtel-Dieu, Paris. 1500. Paris, Musée des Arts Decoratifs, Bibliothèque Nationale. Photo LB 3114, courtesy Giraudon/Art Resource, New York.

Florence of about 1514, depicts women nursing the sick (female only) as the focus of the picture (Fig. 1-17).[26] The presentation is very different from those of northern Europe, however; not only has Pontormo reduced detail to a minimum, he has also made the action mysterious, especially by giving some of the women halos. Since no written documents remain for this painting, it is impossible at the present to read its contents accurately. Nevertheless, it is obvious that the scene differs from northern versions and that it remains unique in Italy.

As we have seen, the Christian nursing type, developed mainly in northern Europe in the fifteenth and early sixteenth centuries, shows a nurse who is neither kin nor servant to the patient, or for that matter to the doctor, although her actions are the very same ones that a wife or a servant might perform. She cares for a person (usually male, I think) in a bed, and that unit may be multiplied to create a hospital ward. She is not represented as the physician's assistant, and priests are more common male presences in these pictures than are doctors.

The emergence of the nun from her cloister and her institutionalized association with nursing and hospitals seem to have begun in western Eu-

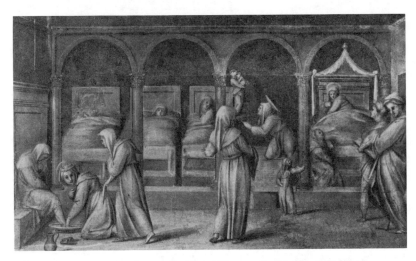

FIGURE 1-17. Pontormo, Story of a Holy Woman (?), Hospital Ward. Ca. 1514.
Florence, Galleria dell'Accademia. Photo 1633, courtesy Alinari/Art Resource,
New York.

rope with the women's religious orders, which served in hospitals during
the twelfth- and thirteenth-century Crusades. The Italian saints, Francis
and Clare, by stressing the public nurturing roles of religious orders during the thirteenth century, contributed to the nun's association with nursing. In the period of increased urbanization and economic expansion in
northern Europe in the fourteenth and fifteenth centuries, the need to care
for the homeless and poor sick of the towns drew the Church into more
and more active competition with the elders of the towns. Both religious
and secular populations were entering the field of social welfare, one as a
matter of Christian duty, the other for the well-being of the town and its
residents.[27] Thus, the social and religious environment produced an interest in and a need for public health care, religion created a population to
serve, and the competition of Church and town produced the patrons to
fund and manage the large city hospitals. All these factors combined with
the new desire for an art whose form and content could imitate the real
secular world. The Christian nursing type grew out of this environment
and reflects its changing social patterns and needs.

An important problem of interpretation is embedded in this analysis of
nursing iconography; nursing sisters seem to be among the first women
shown in Christian art who work with strangers, men as well as women,

outside their own houses. Further, by comparison with later images of nurses, they seem remarkably independent of male physicians. And yet, their activities are exactly the same as those of nonprofessionals, wives and mothers, saints, and women performing acts of mercy. Are we seeing the growth of an iconography of professionalism or a continuation of women's images as domestic nurturers? I think the solution to the problem rests in the Christian theological vision of the hospital. The French called them Hôtels-Dieu, or God's hospices/hostels/homes, and they were tended by God's brides, who cared for His family under His fatherly supervision. Christianity created a synthesis from the nurse as kin and the nurse as public worker; the nursing sister brought this about precisely because she was a holy woman and a servant of Christ. Her independence, her domestic activities, and her public visibility all become understandable and acceptable in this view and keep her from moving outside the bounds of propriety and tradition.

Flemish Art, Seventeenth Century

The last problem I want to consider in this discussion of the artistic and social factors responsible for the creation of nursing iconography concerns the artistic use of the nurse to illustrate social tensions in seventeenth-century Catholic Flanders. I have examined thus far the ancient divisions between public and private in the representation of women as providers of health care, and I have also looked at the religious and artistic synthesis of public and private in the Renaissance creation of an iconography for nursing sisters. In seventeenth-century Flemish art, the Renaissance iconography was used to clarify religious and social relationships for a society that was both intensely religious and intensely secular at the same time. Here, as earlier, the image of the nurse says more about a society and its beliefs than about the nurses themselves.

Flanders's wealth, which came from textiles and trade, supported the arts as well as hospitals, and the country's richest towns kept alive the tradition of the nursing sister in paintings and sculpture in the seventeenth and eighteenth centuries. For the Hospice of Saint Elizabeth in Antwerp, Jacob Jordaens painted a group portrait of nursing sisters at work (Fig. 1-18); for the mental hospital at Gheel, an anonymous artist painted the patients and sisters in the ward; and for the pharmacy of Saint John's

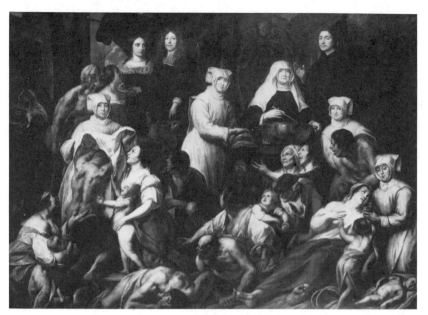

FIGURE I-18. Jacob Jordaens, Antwerp Hospital Sisters. Seventeenth century. Antwerp, Koninklijk Museum voor Schone Kunsten. Photo courtesy Ministerie van de Vlaamse Gemeenschap, Antwerp.

Hospital in Bruges, an anonymous furniture maker carved an oak side-board with sisters nursing and working in the pharmacy (Figs. 1-19, 1-20).[28] In these examples, as in contemporary pictures of Saint Elizabeth or the Seven Works of Mercy, which were still popular in this period, the iconography followed the patterns I discussed above.[29] Styles changed, as did some iconographic elements, such as the addition of a few new medical treatments; now nursing sisters appeared more often in portraits and were often documented as the patrons who paid for nursing pictures.[30] Thus, the images themselves have changed very little, but the conditions in which they were produced and appreciated were different.

The popularity of the scene of sisters nursing the sick in seventeenth-century Flanders seems to depend on its ability to clarify the tensions between Catholic and Protestant, between Church and civil authorities, and between school-educated male physicians and independent female practitioners. In the sixteenth century, Flanders and Holland had separated, no longer to have the same political connections or government or

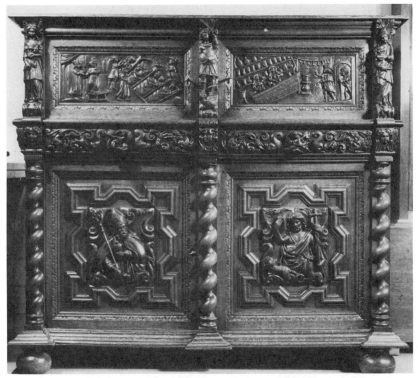

FIGURE 1-19. Anonymous Belgian Cabinetmaker, Carved Sideboard. Seventeenth Century. Bruges, Saint John's Hospital-Memlingmuseum. Photo courtesy Openbaar Centrum voor Maatschappelijk Welzijn, Bruges.

the same religion: Holland became Protestant; Flanders stayed Catholic. Flemish Catholics followed the rulings of the Council of Trent, held by the Church in the 1530s to deal with attacks by reformers like Martin Luther. This Counter-Reformation council reaffirmed the Catholic obligation to perform "good works," the Seven Works of Mercy among them, as a response to the Protestant belief that faith and grace alone were the way to salvation.[31] Flanders may have had a special interest in the representation of good works in art because it had become so pivotal an issue in distinguishing between Catholic Flemish and Protestant Dutch.

The religious hospitals in Flemish towns seem to have been particularly interested, as were the churches, in patronage of works of art that associated Church and charitable activities, part of the ongoing struggle be-

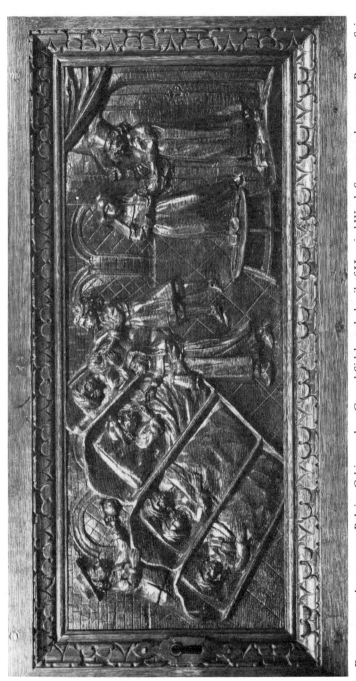

FIGURE 1-20. Anonymous Belgian Cabinetmaker, Carved Sideboard, detail of Hospital Ward. Seventeenth century. Bruges, Saint John's Hospital-Memlingmuseum. Photo courtesy Openbaar Centrum voor Maatschappelijk Welzijn, Bruges.

tween Church and civil authorities for control of charity.[32] The nursing sisters, like Saint Elizabeth and the women in the Seven Works of Mercy pictures, brought to visible form the Catholic ideal, separating it from the Protestant and the secular at the same time.

A further tension was clarified through the iconography of nursing in Counter-Reformation Flanders. There, as in Germany and France, two related social changes were causing crisis—the growth of witch hunts and the increase in the power of secular male physicians. The emphasis on nursing as a right and charitable female religious activity placed it in vivid opposition not only to witchcraft but also to science. In this period, paintings and prints of witches were extremely popular. Franz Francken the Younger's picture *The Witches' Gathering* is a good example of the type in its parody of healing and nursing activities; at the right, a witch even seems to be treating a person with a back ailment (Fig. 1-21). Such images should be seen in relation to the equally great interest in hospital pictures and the Seven Works of Mercy as evidence for a broad concern with women who give both good and evil attention to others.[33] At the same time, we should note that prints, both medical and genre, seem by the seventeenth century to be developing a focus on the male doctor as diagnostician and surgeon; even obstetrical iconography began to incorporate him when the depiction of Caesarian sections grew more popular than midwife-assisted deliveries in art.[34] This is the same historical moment when midwives' instruction books were telling women, as were the new licensing procedures, that they ought to defer to physicians.[35] The scenes of nursing sisters in seventeenth-century Flemish art helped clarify the tensions between secular and religious, between Catholic and Protestant, and between male and female practitioners.[36] The pictures offer answers that are intensely Catholic and that value spiritual and physical nurturance more than scientific and surgical intervention. They all speak through the medium of the nun as good wife and servant of God.

Two main iconographic lines of development, one secular, the other Christian, appear in the representation of women as providers of health care. Antiquity created images of the nursemaid and the midwife, and both were taken over by medieval and later art. What the ancient world could not provide was an imagery of women as nurses for the sick; only Christianity, with its theological synthesis of domestic and public service, was able to provide that. Through the Seven Corporal Works of Mercy, the nursing saint, and the hospital nursing sister, the new synthesis became visible in northern Europe. It served, especially during the Counter-

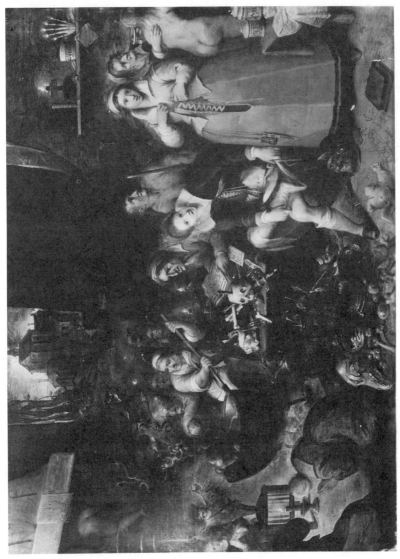

FIGURE 1-21. Franz Francken the Younger, *The Witches' Gathering*. Seventeenth century. Vienna, Kunsthistorisches Museum. Photo courtesy Kunsthistorisches Museum, Vienna.

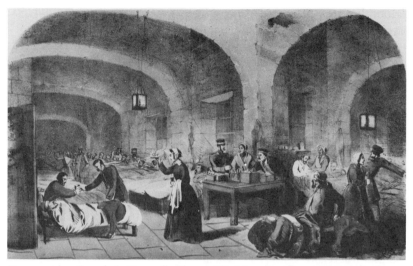

FIGURE 1-22. Joseph A. Benwell, *Florence Nightingale at Scutari*. Nineteenth century. London, Wellcome Institute Library. Photo courtesy Wellcome Institute Library, London.

Reformation, as a way to make visible critical social tensions. Rather than a true iconography of the professional woman, the nurse's image offered a new interpretation of age-old female roles in a Christian context. A later secular age would have to reinterpret that iconography in light of social change before the nurse could begin her struggle to appear as an educated professional.

In this brief survey of a few issues among the many worth considering in an art historical study of nursing, I have focused on classical antiquity and the period from the fifteenth to the seventeenth century in western Europe. I have left out much—the whole world outside of Europe, preclassical and medieval art, and, most significantly for nurses today, art from 1700 on. The period of secularization of nursing iconography begins at that point, moving nurses out of the world of religion and into wage labor and professionalism; by 1850 we are faced with new problems in the creation of images and meanings. Among the many issues left untouched here, we might consider the iconography of woman as "angel in the house" or Florence Nightingale as the lady with the lamp as she appears in a British painting of the later nineteenth century (Fig. 1-22).[37] The changing visual relationship of female nurse and male physician has yet to be fully explored, and the impact on iconography of the changing status of women who worked as nurses in the nineteenth and twentieth centuries needs investigation. To uncover the sources of the white-clad nurse of today's mass media, questions like these need to be studied. What my introductory work has done is to set out the prehistory of today's nursing imagery and to show that contemporary problems of status have their roots in the images of earlier eras. The nurse as saintly domestic is no modern invention.

Notes

1. Previous work on paintings of nurses may be found in Grace Goldin, "A Walk through a Ward of the Eighteenth Century," *Journal of the History of Medicine and Allied Sciences* 22 (April 1967): 121–38; Grace Goldin, "A Painting in Gheel," *Journal of the History of Medicine and Allied Sciences* 26 (October 1971): 400–412; and John D. Thompson and Grace Goldin, *The Hospital: A Social and Architectural History* (New Haven: Yale University Press, 1975), passim.

2. Galen *On Prognosis* 8.1–15, on the cure by a male doctor of the wife of Flavius Boethus; and see also information on the medical profession in the introduction by Owsei Temkin to *Soranus' Gynaecology* (Baltimore: Johns Hopkins Press, 1956), xxxvii.

3. For Greek vase paintings, see Elena Zevi, *Scene di gineceo e scene di idillo nei vasi greci della seconda metà del secolo quinto* (Rome: R. Accademia nazionale dei Lincei, 1938); and Robert F. Sutton, "Interaction between Men and Women Portrayed on Attic Red-figure Pottery" (Ph.D. Diss., University of North Carolina, Chapel Hill, 1981).

4. For female health care personnel in Roman villas, see Columella *De Re Rustica* 12.1.6 and 12.3.7–8. See Livy *Histories* 2.47 and also Franz J. Tritsch, "The Women of Pylos," in *Minoica: Festschrift J. Sundwall,* ed. Ernst Grumach (Berlin: Akademie-Verlag, 1958), 440, n. 68, for women helping to nurse the wounded.

5. For further discussion of the Ostia relief, see Natalie Kampen, *Image and Status* (Berlin: Gebrüder Mann Verlag, 1981), 69–72, 140; for further discussion of the Cypriote terra cotta figurine, see Tones Speteres, *The Art of Cyprus* (New York: Reynal, 1970), 157.

6. For further discussion of the Roman biographical sarcophagus, see Kampen, cat. 25, p. 147; for further discussion of Roman images of nursemaids, see Kampen, 33–44, 146–49.

7. Soranus 1.3–4; for tombstone inscriptions, see *Corpus Inscriptionum Latina-*

rum 6.9477: "Valeria Berecunda [sic], the premier doctor of her region," or *Corpus Inscriptionum Latinarum* 6.9720: "Claudia Trophime the obstetrician"; for legal references, see *Digest* 50.13.1.2: "Governors hear midwives too (in court cases), they also being considered to practice medicine." Translations are mine. For further material on midwives and a few female physicians, see Kampen, 69–72.

8. Sister Mary Rosario, *The Nurse in Greek Life* (Boston: Foreign Language Print Company, 1917), passim; and Kampen, 33–44.

9. Kampen, 41–44; and Alfred Hermann, "Das erste Bad des Heilands und des Helden," *Jahrbuch für Antike und Christentum* 10 (1967): 61–81.

10. Soranus 1.3–4 and 2.4–14, for textual evidence.

11. For discussion of the Vienna manuscript, see Loren MacKinney, *Medical Illustrations in Medieval Manuscripts* (London: Wellcome Historical Medical Library, 1965), no. 92.

12. For an illustration of the Trostbüchle, see Harold Speert, *Iconographia Gyniatrica* (Philadelphia: F. A. Davis, 1973), chap. 4, pl. 13.

13. For further discussion of the ivory, see Hermann, 64–67; for an illustration of the Alexander mosaic, see Maurice Chéhab, "Mosaiques du Liban," *Bulletin du Musée de Beyrouth* 15 (1959): pl. 22; for further discussion of the bath of the infant hero, see Hermann, passim; and Lelia Cracco Ruggini, "Sulla cristianizzazione della cultura pagana," *Athenaeum* 43 (1965): 3–80.

14. For further discussion and for an illustration, see Nancy R. Fabbri and Nina Rutenburg, "The Tabernacle of Orsanmichele in Context," *Art Bulletin* 63 (September 1981): 392–95 and fig. 7.

15. Charles Sterling, *The Hours of Étienne Chevalier* (New York: G. Braziller, 1971); Anonymous Artist of the Upper Rhine, Birth of the Baptist, Musée Unterlinden, Colmar (Speert, chap. 4, pl. 65); see also the motif of the nurse on Italian birth salvers, for example, Paul F. Watson, "A *Desco da Parto* by Bartolomeo di Fruosino," *Art Bulletin* 56 (March 1974): 4–9; as well as Diane Cole Ahl, "Renaissance Birth Salvers and the Richmond *Judgment of Solomon*," *Studies in Iconography* 7–8 (1981–82): 157–74.

16. For an illustration of the fifteenth-century woodcut *The Impatience of the Sick Man* (Paris, Bibliothèque Nationale), see Jean Rousselot, ed., *Medicine in Art* (New York: McGraw-Hill, 1967), 103.

17. Craig Harbison, *The Last Judgment in Sixteenth-Century Northern Europe* (New York: Garland Press, 1976), 106–16.

18. Ibid.

19. For further discussion, see *Rijksmuseum Bulletin* 23 (1976): 203–26.

20. For further examples, see Harbison, 110–11, 277, no. 64.

21. For discussion of the iconography of Saint Elizabeth, see Louis Réau, *Iconographie de l'Art Chrétien: Iconographie des Saints* (Paris: Presses universitaires de France, 1958), 3:417–21, with bibliography and lists of images (incomplete); for discussion of healing saints, see Emil F. Frey, "Saints in Medical History," *Clio Medica* 14 (January 1979): 35–70; for discussion of Cosmas and Damian, see Marie-Louise David-Danel, *Iconographie des saints*

médecins, Côme et Damien (Lille: Morel et Cordurant, 1958); and for illustrations of healing saints, see Roberto Margotta, Illustrated History of Medicine (Feltham: Hamlyn, 1968).

22. Leonhard Küppers, Elisabeth (Recklinghausen: Bongers, 1967), 47.

23. For discussion, see the exhibition catalogue of Sint-Janshospitaal Brugge 1188/ 1976 (Bruges: Commissie van Openbaar Onderstand van Brugge, 1976), 1:40, fig. 8.

24. For illustration and discussion, see Dix siècles d'histoire hospitalière parisienne: L'Hôtel-Dieu de Paris (Paris: Musée de l'Assistance Publique, 1961), 37–41; and Musée de l'Assistance Publique de Paris (Paris: Musée de l'Assistance Publique, 1981), no. 5.

25. For illustrations, see MacKinney, 6–7, fig. 3; or Domenico di Bartolo, fifteenth-century fresco, Hospital of Santa Maria della Scala, Siena, in Rousselot, 104.

26. For discussion, see Sidney J. Freedberg, Painting in the High Renaissance in Rome and Florence (Cambridge: Harvard University Press, 1961), 1:244–45.

27. Vern and Bonnie Bullough, The Care of the Sick (London: C. Helm, 1979), 38ff.; Timothy S. Miller, "The Knights of St. John and the Hospitals of the Latin West," Speculum 53 (October 1978): 709–33; and on the relationship between secular and religious authority over charity, see John Baptist Knipping, Iconography of the Counter-Reformation in the Netherlands (Nieuwkoop: De Graaf, 1974), 2:328–32.

28. For discussion of Jordaens's painting, see the exhibition catalogue Jordaens in Belgisch Bezit (Antwerp: Ministerie van Nederlandse Cultuur, 1978), no. 39; for further discussion of the Gheel painting, see Goldin, "A Painting in Gheel," passim; and for further discussion of the sideboard, see Valentin Vermeersch, Brugges Kunstbezit (Bruges: Desclée de Brouwer, 1973), 2:147–51. See also eighteenth-century examples such as Beerblock's representation of the ward at Bruges's Saint John's Hospital of ca. 1778 (for discussion of it, see Goldin, "Walk through a Ward") or the little-known paintings of the sisters of Port Royal des Champs by Madeleine de Boulogne in the Versailles Museum (for an illustration, see Maxime Laignel-Lavastine, Histoire générale de la médecine . . . (Paris: Albin Michel, 1949), chap. 3, pl. 254.

29. For an illustration of Martin Pepyn's Saint Elizabeth Altarpiece, see Reginald H. Wilenski, Flemish Painters (New York: Viking, 1960), vol. 2, pl. 569; for discussion and an illustration of David Teniers the Younger's Seven Works of Mercy, see Jane P. Davidson, David Teniers the Younger (Boulder: Westview Press, 1979), 17, 19–20, and pl. 3; for discussion of contemporary Flemish paintings and prints of the Seven Works, see also Knipping, 328–32.

30. See the exhibition catalogue of Sint-Janshospitaal Brugge 1188/1976, 2:44–57; and the fifteenth-century predecessor, Hans Memlinc's portraits of nuns on the Shrine of Saint Ursula, 6.

31. Knipping, 328–32.

32. Ibid.

33. On witchcraft and its relationship to medicine in this period, see Thomas R.

Forbes, *The Midwife and the Witch* (New Haven: Yale University Press, 1966); Barbara Ehrenreich and Deirdre English, *Witches, Midwives, and Nurses: A History of Women Healers* (Old Westbury, N.Y.: Feminist Press, 1973); and H. C. Eric Midelfort, *Witch Hunting in Southwestern Germany, 1562–1684* (Palo Alto: Stanford University Press, 1972), 187, on the prominence of midwives in the lists of women taken as witches.

34. This impression has not, to my knowledge, been confirmed by any study to quantify the images. The historical phenomenon is discussed in a specific case in Esther Fischer-Homberger, "Hebammen und Hymen," *Sudhoffs Archiv* 61 (January 1977): 75–94.

35. Thomas G. Benedek, "The Changing Relationship between Midwives and Physicians during the Renaissance," *Bulletin of the History of Medicine* 51 (Winter 1977): 550–64.

36 On seventeenth- and eighteenth-century medical staff relations, see Louis S. Greenbaum, "Nurses and Doctors in Conflict: Piety and Medicine in the Paris Hôtel-Dieu on the Eve of the French Revolution," *Clio Medica* 13 (May 1978): 247–67.

37. I have seen only a small part of an unpublished manuscript of 1973 by J. W. Forsaith, "The Lady with a Lamp," for which reference I thank the staff of the Wellcome Institute of the History of Medicine.

Rima D. Apple

2. Image or Reality?
Photographs in the History of Nursing

Lady with the lamp, ministering angel, Sairey Gamp: such literary images create in our minds pictures of nurses, pictures that reinforce stereotypes and make history more concrete and more immediate. Literature, however, is not the only source of graphic portrayals of nurses. Scholars frequently exploit the vivifying effects of visual images in historical presentations. Authors and publishers insert eye-catching illustrations in textbooks; lecturers engage the attention of students with pictures and slides. And photographs, since they appear to represent "reality," are often the preferred illustrative form.

Recently, researchers have begun to look beyond photographs as simple illustrations and to approach these images as complex primary source documents for historical analysis. Photography discloses physical details and textures only implied in written and oral sources. Relationships among people and between people and institutions not discussed explicitly in other types of sources frequently appear dramatically in photographic images. Furthermore, a photograph used to exemplify one point or a generally accepted historical interpretation may at the same time inform us about allied issues. As with analyses of other sources, photographic research is not an end in itself but rather an approach to historical study with which we can enhance our understanding of the past.

The attributes of photographic research make it especially valuable and applicable to women's history in general and to the history of nursing in particular. Many aspects of these histories never appear in more traditional source materials. In printed sources, for example, nurses are usually seen through the eyes of physicians and hospital administrators, who viewed the nurse as subordinate to the (male) physician, or of nursing leaders, who sought to promote the professionalization of nursing.

Focusing on the image of hospital nurses in the late nineteenth and early twentieth centuries, I examine in this essay the use of photographs as illustrations and as objects of historical research. Photographic evidence confirms both the prescriptive images of nurses found in other contemporary sources and the descriptive images developed in current histories of nursing. Moreover, it documents differences between the idealized views and the concrete experiences of hospital life. Significantly, it reveals events not mentioned in other sources. Before addressing the particular question of the image of hospital nurses at the turn of the century, however, I must discuss some problems encountered in this mode of historical inquiry.

Compared with the plethora of other materials from the period, the unevenness of the photographic record is striking. Some photographs are reproduced in contemporary and historical publications; others are found in iconographic and institutional archives. But since archivists and librarians traditionally have been more concerned with written sources, photographic collections often are inadequately preserved and inconsistently catalogued. Many photographs remain in private hands, either as collectors' items or as family mementos, making them difficult for historians to locate and study.[1]

Furthermore, while certain themes were popular photographic subjects, other relatively common areas of life were only infrequently photographed. For example, only a small number of private-duty and home-care nursing photographs exist. Yet most nurses at the turn of the century were employed as private-duty nurses, often in the homes of middle-class and upper-class families. Several factors undoubtedly contributed to the scarcity of such photographs. The practice itself was so commonplace that few people probably thought to record it in photographs. Also, home care usually concerned situations that the families involved would prefer to forget, not to relive pleasantly through photographs. And unlike the numerous schools and hospitals inspired to memorialize their activities in photographs, few visiting nurses' associations and similar groups existed at the turn of the century. Thus, what photographic evidence we have must be analyzed cautiously and placed in context.[2]

When writers and teachers use photographs as "mirrors of reality" or "windows through which we view our past," they sometimes ignore the important questions of whose windows and what reality. Frequently missing from the historical records is any mention of why the photograph was taken and how it was used. With information about, for example, who commissioned the picture and for what purpose, it is possible to evaluate how "candid" a reflection of "reality" the photograph portrays and the relative importance of the scene photographed. Consequently, photographs reproduced with accompanying text in, say, annual reports can sometimes be more useful to researchers than original prints or negatives separated from supporting documentation. Family photo albums are another case in point. People generally photographed significant domestic events, not day-to-day affairs. An anniversary party, a homecoming, a vacation trip, seen in the context of an album collection, suggest what the family deemed important and memorable; viewed as isolated photographs they would tell much less.

Seeing the camera as a neutral observer, we tend to accept photographs as "truer" representations of "real life" than other, more subjective visual forms such as paintings. After all, it is said, a camera cannot lie; it can only preserve what it sees, providing an image of neither more nor less than appears before it (unless the negative is retouched). Yet the same conscious and unconscious biases that affect written and oral sources influence photographs. Photographers position cameras, select the frame (what to include and what to exclude), and even manipulate persons and things to produce a desired image. The mere presence of a photographer can modify a scene; for instance, participants' awareness of the camera may alter their stance, expression, or action.

Despite these limitations and difficulties, photographic research is still a particularly fruitful line of historical investigation. Acquaintance with secondary and supplemental sources alleviates the danger of unwarranted generalizations based on unrepresentative samples of images, as with hospital and private-duty nursing. Familiarity with other, similar photographs helps to place an otherwise unidentified image in a meaningful context. Even the acknowledged bias of the camera assists the historian by suggesting the quality or image that the photographer or participants wanted to preserve.[3] Beginning with a carefully posed, representative portrait and proceeding through to an anomalous, "candid" photograph, I will demonstrate in this study how photographic analyses can inform our understanding of turn-of-the-century nurses and nursing.

In 1898, Jane Hodson, graduate of the New York Hospital Training School and nursing director at the State Hospital, Fountain Springs, Pennsylvania, edited the volume *How to Become a Trained Nurse*. The publication was directed to young women interested in a career in nursing and contained articles on nursing, entries on training schools in North America, and numerous photographs. The tone of the book was both inspirational and practical. Each school's description included information about the size of the hospital and departments in it, the number of students and graduates, length of training, type and extent of instruction, and "last, but not least, the important question as to whether she [the student nurse] may expect to have a room to herself or share it with other nurses, as is sometimes the case even in the best hospitals."[4] This quotation conveys the editor's ideas about what class of woman nursing should attract. Who, in the 1890s, would expect or aspire to her own room at training school? A respectable, refined woman, perhaps the daughter of a well-to-do or middle-class family, or one who saw entry into the nursing profession as a means of attaining middle-class status. Readers concerned with class size, instructional modes, and the like were probably practical-minded women interested in their professional preparation.

Photographs reproduced in the book also evoke this interpretation of Hodson's ideal nurse. One can sense it in the portrait of a head nurse, student nurse, and probationer at Boston City Hospital (Fig. 2-1), which also substantiates other information of turn-of-the-century nurses. Their dress, while not necessarily serviceable on the wards, was "proper." Their demeanors suggest that these poised women saw their roles as professionals; their careers represented more to them than mere paid employment. And their pose gives visual evidence of the oft-discussed hierarchical relationships within the hospital nursing staff. Each woman appears to have, and to know, her place. Befitting her rank, the head nurse is seated in the foreground; standing slightly behind her is the pupil; behind both of them and somewhat to the side is the probationer, a woman not yet fully admitted to the training school.

Other books from the same era provide additional photographic evidence of contemporaries' idealized image of nurses, but they also raise questions. Little is known about the impetus to publish *Prominent Physicians, Surgeons, Medical Institutions of Cook County,* which describes the various health care facilities and schools in Chicago in 1899.[5] Internal evidence suggests that it was a promotional volume designed to glorify the medical care available in the city. Entries for each institution include information about its structure and accommodations, the number of patients treated, and its staff, and they frequently declare, as in the entry for Provident Hospital, "the management most respectfully invites the attention of surgeons and physicians."[6] Provident established a nurse training school soon after its founding in the early 1890s. A photograph of a nurses' class (Fig. 2-2) accompanied the article describing Provident.

The classroom setting conveys the image of nurse as educated woman.

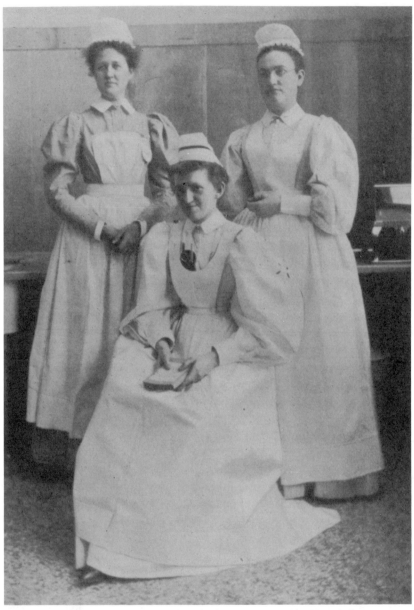

FIGURE 2-1. Head nurse, pupil, and probationer, Boston City Hospital, 1896. From Jane Hodson, ed., *How to Become a Trained Nurse: A Manual of Information in Detail* (New York: William Abbatt, 1898), n.p.

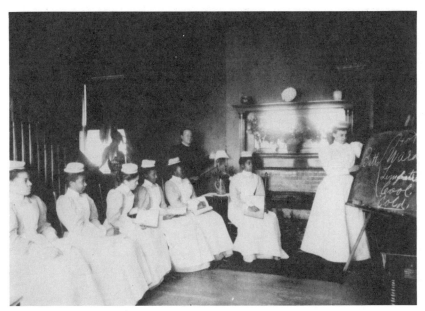

FIGURE 2-2. Nurses' class, Provident Hospital and Training School, Chicago, 1899. From *Prominent Physicians, Surgeons, Medical Institutions of Cook County* (Chicago: Redheffer Art Publishing Company, 1899), n.p.

Since students are attending lectures and taking notes, it seems reasonable to assume that pupils could at minimum read and write. From the photograph it is not possible to deduce how much classroom instruction the women received, but inclusion of this scene implies the significance contemporaries placed on the educational component of the nurse's image. The contrast between the students, all of whom are black (the school prided itself on giving "the opportunity for a life work to many young colored women by opening to them a profession"[7]) and the white nursing instructor at the chalkboard is interesting. Also, there is another white woman standing in the background, possibly the superintendent or the matron. Does this photograph exemplify racial beliefs superimposed on the hierarchy of the nursing staff? While showing what contemporaries considered a positive image of nursing students, this photograph leads to further questions about the status of various groups within the nursing profession.[8]

Imagery such as that found in *How to Become a Trained Nurse* and *Prominent Physicians, Surgeons, Medical Institutions of Cook County* abounds in

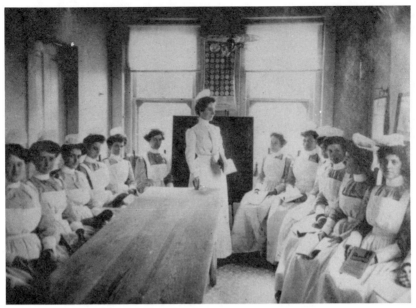

FIGURE 2-3. Nurses' class, Saint Joseph's Hospital, Atlanta, 1906. Photo courtesy Saint Joseph's Hospital Archives, Atlanta, Georgia.

books and journals. Archival sources hold additional examples in print and negative form. A 1906 classroom photograph from Saint Joseph's Hospital, Atlanta (Fig. 2-3), expresses the "book learning" aspect of nursing instruction. The photographer's impact on the picture is evident. Though the people in the nurses' class at Provident Hospital (Fig. 2-2) were undoubtedly aware of the camera, they are posed in a realistic classroom situation. On the other hand, many of the students in this photograph are looking at the camera, not at their books or their teacher. The instructor herself appears to be gazing off at some distant point. A more practical classroom structure would have the students seated at the table; probably they moved their chairs back for the photograph. Several students are placed behind the teacher, an awkward position for instruction. Lacking additional information, I can only speculate on the reasons behind this posed scene: perhaps the photographer felt that a rearrangement of the seating would result in a better picture; possibly a school manager wanted a photograph showing the faces and uniforms of the students. Regardless of why the scene was manipulated or who was responsible, the photo-

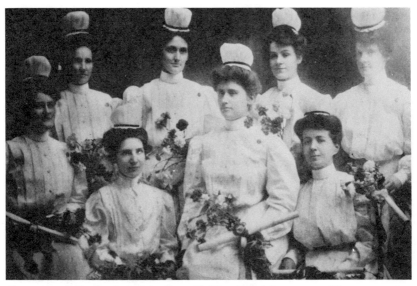

FIGURE 2-4. Graduation, Saint Joseph's Hospital, Atlanta, 1906. Photo courtesy Saint Joseph's Hospital Archives, Atlanta, Georgia.

graph is useful in illustrating contemporaries' views of nurses as educated women.

Another example, a 1906 graduation portrait from Saint Joseph's Hospital, Atlanta (Fig. 2-4), brings into sharp relief the contrast between the ideals of nurses' professionalism and their femininity. Dressed in their crisp white uniforms, proudly displaying their caps and pins, the women appear poised and confident; they have completed their training and are prepared to embark on their chosen careers. On the other hand, the bouquets seem to say that these nurses are not merely professionals; they also are women who remember and celebrate their culture's concept of femininity. To many commentators and nurses themselves, nursing represented an extension of women's roles in the family and in the community, and womanliness was one of the most important characteristics of a good nurse. This graduation picture successfully combines the hard (efficiency) model with the softer (womanly) aspects of nursing.

Do the flowers represent more than femininity? Carrying bouquets is also symbolic of class, reminiscent of debutantes and balls. Did the graduates consider their bouquets status symbols? If so, do the flowers signify the women's own class or the class to which they aspired? Though pre-

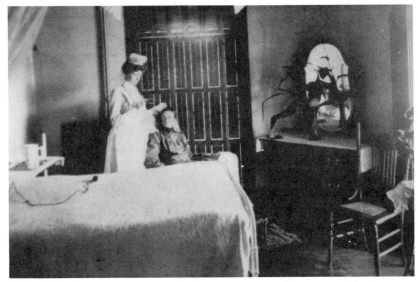

FIGURE 2-5. Private room, Saint Joseph's Hospital, Atlanta, 1903. Photo courtesy Saint Joseph's Hospital Archives, Atlanta, Georgia.

senting a stereotypical view of nurses, this photograph raises many such questions.

Thus far, I have shown consciously structured and posed photographs focused on the nurses themselves. These pictures present views of nurses that contemporaries chose to memorialize: the poise, the professionalism, the education, the womanliness of nurses. Historians can draw significant insights from other photographs that at first glance appear to involve nurses only peripherally. Not that such photographs are any less posed than the previous examples; they often were carefully arranged. However, since they contain unexceptional, accepted aspects of nursing, such pictures denote more clearly the actual position and work of nurses and, perhaps, come closer to expressing the reality of nurses' experiences.

Take, for example, a photograph of a private room, reproduced in the 1903 annual report of Saint Joseph's Hospital, Atlanta (Fig. 2-5). At the turn of the century, hospital administrators promoted the "homeliness" of their institutions and the availability of nursing care to attract middle- and upper-class patients. The 1903 report declared: "When a patient arrives at 'St. Joseph's' he is made to feel at *home*. Every detail that will add to his comfort and pleasure is promptly attended to."[9] (Stress in the original.)

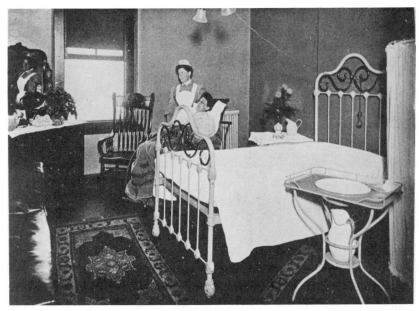

FIGURE 2-6. Private room, Old Michael Reese Hospital, Chicago, ca. 1885–1905. Photo courtesy Michael Reese Hospital and Medical Center Archives, Chicago, Illinois.

The photograph confirms the text's claim: rugs, mirror and dresser, flowers give the room a "home-like" atmosphere. Moreover, combining the emphasis on prompt attention to "comfort and pleasure" with the picture of the nurse standing behind the patient,[10] viewers are forced to consider how much nurses acted as medical attendants and how much they functioned as servants.

Saint Joseph's was not unique. Photographs from other institutions substantiate the servantlike position of hospital nurses. A private room at Old Michael Reese Hospital, Chicago, ca. 1885–1905 (Fig. 2-6), also shows the domestic furnishings, the flowers, and a nurse similarly posed behind the patient. The concept of nurse-as-servant generated from these and other pictures strengthens the conclusions current in today's historiography that emphasize the housekeeping and domestic aspects of nursing in the late nineteenth and early twentieth centuries.

In addition, the photographic record supports the view of nurses as "handmaidens" or servants to physicians, imagery popular in contem-

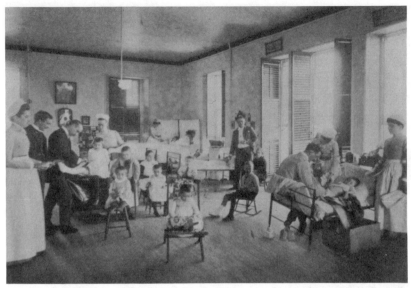

FIGURE 2-7. "Morning Rounds," Children's Ward, Bellevue Hospital, New York, 1898. From Jane Hodson, ed., *How to Become a Trained Nurse: A Manual of Information in Detail* (New York: William Abbatt, 1898), n.p.

poraries' discussions of nursing and in current histories of nursing. "Rounds," one of the most important hospital activities shared by nurses and physicians, followed definite procedures. Typical of the era, Luther Hospital, Eau Claire, Wisconsin, demanded in its "Rules for Nurses" that the head nurse shall:

> make the rounds with the attendants, receive all orders and prescriptions in the giver's handwriting in a book kept for that purpose and see that such orders are promptly and carefully carried out. . . .[11]

There are no photographs of daily rounds at Luther Hospital, but pictures from other institutions document this activity.

Hodson reproduced "Morning Rounds" at the children's ward of Bellevue Hospital, New York (Fig. 2-7), in her volume, obviously to illustrate the work prospective nurses could expect to pursue in their chosen profession. Though the children and at least one physician look directly at the photographer, the nurses seem to be assiduously avoiding the camera. Per-

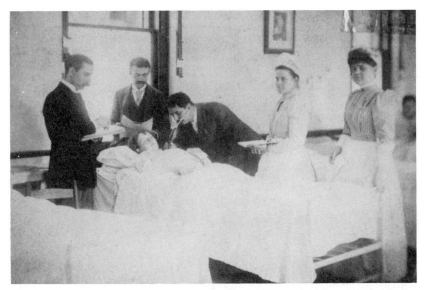

FIGURE 2-8. Rounds, Bellevue Hospital, New York, 1891. Photo courtesy New York University Medical Center Archives, New York, New York.

haps they knew that this photograph would be used to promote nursing and they wished to show nurses as conscientious workers. At any rate, they apparently have taken to heart Rule 19 of Luther Hospital's regulations for nurses:

> Nurses will bear in mind that while they are at all times to be polite and courteous, their relation with the internes, attendants and patients must be strictly professional. . . .[12]

The "help-meet" aspect of nursing is even more distinct in a similar, unpublished photograph taken at the same institution a few years earlier (Fig. 2-8). In this case, the physicians are carefully observing the patient and the nurses are glancing at the camera. The women's different uniforms and their positions relative to the patient and physicians suggest once again the hierarchical structure of the nursing staff. The more senior of the two, dressed all in white and holding a book, stands nearest the doctors; possibly she is a head nurse. Since a physician is writing in one book, most likely the patient's record, the nurse's book is probably for the pre-

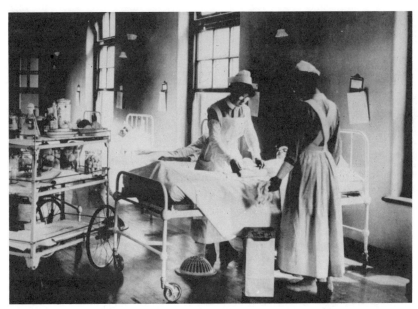

FIGURE 2-9. Collecting soiled dressings, Pennsylvania Hospital, Philadelphia, ca. 1900–1920. Photo courtesy Pennsylvania Hospital Archives, Philadelphia, Pennsylvania.

vious or next patient to be examined. If there were more documentation on the photograph—who took it, who saved it, and why—historians might go further in their analysis. As it is, comparisons with other photographs and their knowledge of the relationships among nurses and between nurses and physicians allow them to place this picture in the context of the history of nursing.

Photographs such as those in Figures 2-7 and 2-8 are also helpful reminders of the significant role nurses played in day-to-day hospital care. Much of the nurse's work undoubtedly involved mundane, dirty, and arduous tasks; yet few photographs remain, if they ever existed, of these aspects of a nurse's life. The paucity of such pictures and the consequent inability to draw conclusions from comparative analyses make the historian even more dependent on supporting documentation, which, unfortunately, is frequently unavailable.

A good case in point is the photograph taken at Pennsylvania Hospital, Philadelphia, sometime during the first two decades of this century (Fig. 2-9). Two nurses, possibly students judging from their dress, are changing

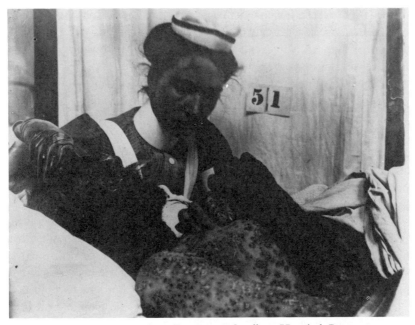

FIGURE 2-10. Nurse and patient, Emergency Smallpox Hospital, Boston, 1902. Photo courtesy The Francis A. Countway Library of Medicine, Boston, Massachusetts.

a ward patient's bandages. Was it usual for two nurses to work together like this? Is one nurse instructing the other? How "natural" or "artificial" is the scene? The light shining through the windows, the gleam of the floors, the location of the medicine cart, which balances the left side of the photograph, all suggest that the photographer carefully arranged and timed the scene. Not that the artificiality of the photograph necessarily negates the "reality" of the work. But if more were known about the photograph, why it was taken and to what uses it was put, the typicality of this version of the nurse's daily work could perhaps be determined.

There is a little more information about the next photograph, part of a clinical record of a patient at the Smallpox Hospital in Boston in 1902 (Fig. 2-10). The physician-in-charge was interested in the patient and the course of the disease, hence the focus on the victim. The nurse appears totally involved with her patient and unaware of the camera; her concern is evident as she seeks to soothe him with her gloved hand on his forehead. Other photographs in this series show her bathing the patient, swabbing his pustulous encrusted eyelids. No doubt untold numbers of nurses performed such tasks in hospitals all over the country; probably a major portion of their work with patients consisted of comforting and providing emotional support. The extant photographic record, however, gives few instances of these aspects of nursing.

In light of the meager sample of photographs depicting routine ward-patient care, the number of surgery pictures is all the more pronounced. Physicians and hospital administrators used photography to capitalize on the impressive advances made in surgery and the dramatic impact of surgery scenes. They frequently reproduced photographs of operating theaters, surgical equipment, and surgery in their reports and promotional publications. Hospital archives and scrapbooks preserve other, unpublished examples of surgical scenes.

Despite the constraints of its hierarchical structure and its subservient position to the medical profession, nursing at the turn of the century, most historians would agree, did not comprise a limited or even distinctive sphere of clearly defined skills. Nurses engaged in an extremely wide range of activities. Although the dearth of ward-work photographs does not allow direct observation of the nurses' varied housekeeping and medical duties, samples drawn from the relatively vast number of unpublished and published surgical photographs show quite clearly that nurses participated in and undertook an amazing array of tasks.

Two representative photographs dated 1903 (Figs. 2-11, 2-12) present the common view of nurses assisting in surgery. The arrangement of both scenes draws the viewer's eye to the surgical procedure itself; the surgeons and anesthetists are of paramount importance. In the photograph from Saint Joseph's Hospital, Atlanta (Fig. 2-11), the nurses appear to be awaiting the physicians' orders. Similarly, in the photograph from Hotel Dieu, El Paso (Fig. 2-12), the doorway seems to frame the physicians in the surgical area and to place the nurses on a plane subsidiary to the major focus of the photograph. Interestingly, the nurses at Saint Joseph's stand on each side of the operating table, their positions giving no indication about their possibly different duties; the placement of the nurses at Hotel Dieu suggests a chain of command according to which the Sister passes the physicians' requests on to the lay nurses working at the table. Both pictures depict nurses in somewhat passive, reactive roles and not intimately connected with the surgery.

How realistic are these pictures of early twentieth-century surgery? Was the photographer present during the actual surgical procedure or was the

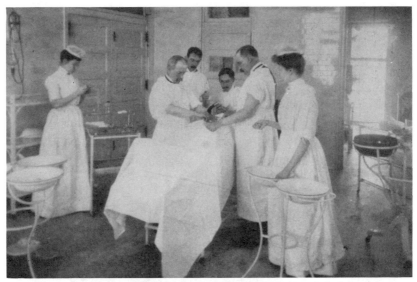

FIGURE 2-11. Nurses assisting in surgery, Saint Joseph's Hospital, Atlanta, 1903. Photo courtesy Saint Joseph's Hospital Archives, Atlanta, Georgia.

FIGURE 2-12. Nurses assisting in surgery, Hotel Dieu, El Paso, 1903. Photo courtesy Hotel Dieu Medical Center Archives, El Paso, Texas.

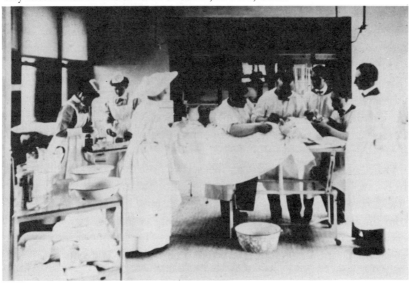

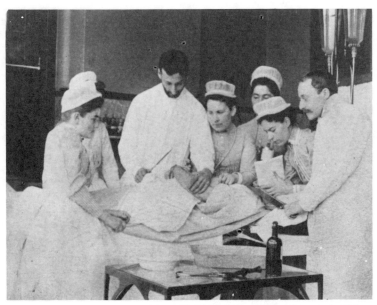

FIGURE 2-13. Operating room with staff, Old Michael Reese Hospital, Chicago, ca. 1890. Photo courtesy Michael Reese Hospital and Medical Center Archives, Chicago, Illinois.

photograph arranged and shot before the operation began? The location and stance of the physicians imply some rearrangement of the scenes for the camera, especially in Figure 2-12, where the observing physician on the right could be expected to be closer to the field of operation. Perhaps the photograph was intended to display the operating room facilities rather than to show an operation. Without knowing the degree to which the photographer may have manipulated the scene, and why, the "reality" of the nurses' auxiliary status in them can still be accepted because these photographs and many others like them depict nurses in the stereotypical role of physicians' "handmaidens."

Other photographs contradict this servile posture and tell of nurses actively involved in surgical procedures. In a photograph taken at Old Michael Reese Hospital, Chicago, in 1890, the nurses are not standing back from the operating table (Fig. 2-13). They are beside the physicians, observing the operation and holding the patient. This scrapbook photograph carries the caption "Operating Room," a fairly limited description of the scene. Since the caption does not mention the operating room attendants, it is possible that at this time nurses at Michael Reese commonly partici-

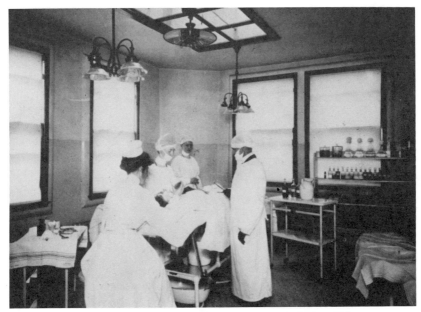

FIGURE 2-14. Nurse anesthetizing patient, Luther Hospital, Eau Claire, 1908. Photo courtesy Luther Hospital, Medical Library, Eau Claire, Wisconsin.

pated in surgery and that their presence, therefore, called for no particular comment. Such a supposition, of course, demands additional evidence. The work of at least one of the nurses in the photograph, the anesthetist, was not unusual.

Extant photographs attest to the frequent employment of nurse-anesthetists in the late nineteenth and early twentieth centuries. In a photograph from 1908 taken at Luther Hospital, Eau Claire, Wisconsin, the surgeons are posed beside the operating table as the nurse anesthetizes the patient (Fig. 2-14). The composition of the scene suggests that she is not on an equal footing with the surgeons: her back is to the camera, perhaps so the photograph more clearly shows the physicians; her dress is distinctly different from theirs—no head-covering, no face-mask, no surgical gown, and possibly no gloves. The separation between the nurse-anesthetist and the surgeons reflects contemporaries' views of anesthesia, which had not yet developed into a medical specialty. For a nurse, surgeons declared, anesthesia was "a stepping-stone to something better than she had originally chosen, a higher and more dignified position. . . ."[13]

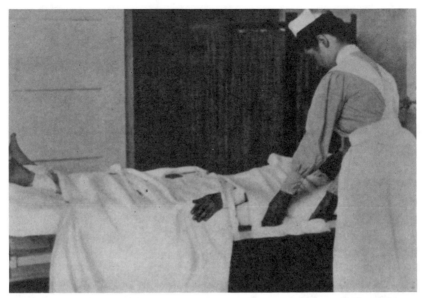

FIGURE 2-15. Postoperative care, 1912. From L. R. G. Crandon and Albert Ehrenfried, *Surgical After-Treatment: A Manual of the Conduct of Surgical Convalescence,* 2d ed. (Philadelphia: W. B. Saunders, 1912), 32. Reprinted with permission
of W. B. Saunders.

For a medical practitioner, the same occupation represented "scientific
narrowness and lack of opportunity for distinction and income," which
therefore did not attract the "man of high grade of intelligence, with a
well-grounded medical and surgical education. . . ."[14] This dual standard
signified that although a nurse-anesthetist might hold a prestigious position vis-à-vis nursing, she in no way acquired the status of a physician.
Moreover, surgeons preferred a nurse-anesthetist because she would continue to care for the patient in the recovery room (Fig. 2-15), where "vigi-
lance is necessary, not only to prevent the unconscious patient from
swallowing his tongue or choking in mucus or vomitus, but also from
injuring himself in delirium, or from removing or displacing his dressing."[15] In other words, unlike physician-anesthetists, nurse-anesthetists as
nurses would take over the arduous, and in some respects menial, though
possibly lifesaving, aspects of after-surgery care.

Either as assistants or anesthetists, nurses in these surgery photographs
acted under physicians; they remained true to our historical concept of
nursing as subservient to the medical profession. Given this commonly

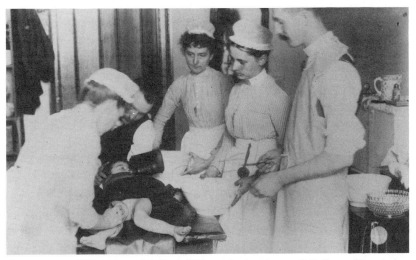

FIGURE 2-16. "Osteotomy for Genu-Valgum by head nurse," Bellevue Hospital, New York, 1890–91. Photo courtesy the Edward G. Miner Library, University of Rochester School of Medicine and Dentistry, Rochester, New York.

accepted view, the next photograph (Fig. 2-16) is all the more arresting. Mounted in a scrapbook inscribed "To Kittie L. Pond, Compliments of J. L. Whitcomb, M.D., Bellevue Hospital [New York], Christmas 1890–1891," the photograph is plainly captioned "Osteotomy for Genu-Valgum by head nurse." Careful examination of the picture confirms that the nurse on the left is not the anesthetist: she is not handing equipment to a surgeon; she is holding an instrument, possibly a scalpel, and is about to begin a procedure, probably an incision in the child's leg. How are we to evaluate this scene?

The scant information available raises more questions than it answers. Whitcomb interned at Bellevue in 1890 and 1891.[16] Was he the photographer? Is he in the picture? Did he commission the photograph? What was his relationship to Pond? Was she the head nurse? The woman prepared to make the incision does appear several other times in the album, but with no more identification than head nurse. The number of photographs of the head nurse and the album's inscription lead me to conjecture that Pond was the head nurse, but Bellevue's records are incomplete, and I cannot confirm this assumption.

Naming the nurse would still leave the important puzzle of the scene. Did the head nurse regularly operate? From historians' knowledge of nursing and surgical history, this explanation is very unlikely. The photograph might commemorate an unusual case. Or the operation might have been posed for the camera and never actually been completed by the nurse. Both scenarios are possible. Accepting the former hypothesis would force the conclusion that the occupational sphere of nurses in the 1890s was much broader than previously believed. The latter suggests the participants recognized the status of surgery and wanted at least one nurse to adopt some of its mystique. The story will probably never be known, but this photograph with all its unanswered and unanswerable questions forces reevaluation of some views of nursing.

As the sixteen examples in this essay demonstrate, historical studies can gain much from photographic research.[17] Photographs are powerful illustrative tools. When discussed in their original context, they clarify insights into contemporaries' views of nurses: refined, educated women, confident in their choice of career, who served both their patients and physicians. Moreover, carefully examined photographs provide the tools to qualify the idealized image of the era. Such pictures evoke a sense of daily life not conveyed by written sources and help make the work of the hospital nurse on the ward and in the operating room more explicit. Anomalous photographs compel historians to question anew commonly accepted interpretations. While in some instances reinforcing stereotypes and substantiating contemporary historiographic conclusions, photographic analysis highlights important areas for further inquiry, leads to research that can expand historians' understanding, and may reformulate historical images of the hospital nurse.

Notes

1. The citations to photographs in this essay indicate the variety of published and archival sources for historical medical photographs. For a more extensive listing, see Rima D. Apple, comp., *Illustrated Catalogue of the Slide Archive of Historical Medical Photographs at Stony Brook, Center for Photographic Images of Medicine and Health Care* (Westport, Conn.: Greenwood Press, 1984).
2. Basic historical sources that provide a context for evaluating photographic evidence include Nancy Tomes, "'Little World of Our Own': The Pennsylvania Hospital Training School for Nurses, 1895–1907," *Journal of the History of Medicine and Allied Sciences* 33 (October 1978): 507–30; Barbara Melosh, *"The Physicians' Hand": Work Culture and Conflict in American Nursing* (Philadelphia: Temple University Press, 1982); Susan Reverby, *Ordered to Care: The Dilemma of American Nursing* (New York: Cambridge University Press,

1987). In addition, see Philip A. Kalisch and Beatrice J. Kalisch, *The Advance of American Nursing* (Boston: Little, Brown, 1978), which is also a good example of an illustrated textbook.

3. For further discussion of these points, see Marsha Peters and Bernard Mergen, "'Doing the Rest': The Uses of Photographs in American Studies," *American Quarterly* 29 (Bibliography Issue 1977): 280–303; Michael Thomason, "The Magic Image Revisited: The Photograph as a Historical Source," *Alabama Review* 31 (April 1978): 83–91; Walter Rundell, Jr., "Photographs as Historical Evidence: Early Texas Oil," *American Archivist* 41 (October 1978): 373–98; Alan Trachtenberg, "Introduction: Photographs as Symbolic History," in *The American Image: Photographs from the National Archives, 1860–1960,* United States National Archives and Records Service (New York: Pantheon, 1979), ix–xxxii; James West Davidson and Mark Hamilton Lytle, "The Mirror with a Memory: Photographic Evidence and the Urban Scene," in *After the Fact: The Art of Historical Detection* (New York: Alfred A. Knopf, 1981), 2:205–39; James S. Terry, Antol Herskovitz, and Daniel M. Fox, "Photographs Tell More Than Meets the Eye," *Journal of Biological Photography* 48 (July 1980): 111–15; Madelyn Moeller, "Photography and History: Using Photographs in Interpreting our Cultural Past," *Journal of American Culture* 6 (Spring 1983): 3–17; Cathy Slusser, "Women of Tampa Bay: A Photo Essay," *Tampa Bay History* 5 (Fall/Winter 1984): 47–63; Jill Gates Smith, "Women in Health Care Delivery: The Histories of Women, Medicine and Photography," *Caduceus: A Museum Quarterly for the Health Sciences* 1 (Winter 1985): 1–4; James S. Terry, "Dissecting Room Portraits: Decoding an Underground Genre," *History of Photography* 7 (April–June 1983): 96–98; and Hilary Russell, "Reflections of an Image Finder: Some Problems and Suggestions for Picture Research," *Material History Bulletin* 20 (Fall 1984): 79–83.

4. Jane Hodson, "Preface," in *How to Become a Trained Nurse: A Manual of Information in Detail,* ed. Jane Hodson (New York: William Abbatt, 1898), n.p.

5. *Prominent Physicians, Surgeons, Medical Institutions of Cook County* (Chicago: Redheffer Art Publishing Company, 1899).

6. Ibid., n.p.

7. Ibid.

8. For a history of Provident Hospital and Training School, see Patricia Ellen Sloan, "A History of the Establishment and Early Development of Selected Nurse Training Schools for Afro-Americans: 1886–1906" (Ed.D. Diss., Teachers College, Columbia University, 1977). Other recent scholarship on the history of black nurses includes Patricia E. Sloan, "Black Hospitals and Nurse Training Schools: The Formative Years, 1880–1900" (Paper presented at the Fifth Berkshire Conference on the History of Women, June 1981); Darlene Clark Hine, "The Ethel Johns Report: Black Women in the Nursing Profession, 1925," *Journal of Negro History* 67 (Fall 1982): 212–28; and Darlene Clark Hine, "'They Shall Mount Up with Wings as Eagles': Historical Images of Black Nurses, 1890–1950," in this volume, chap. 8, pp. 177–96.

9. Saint Joseph's Hospital, *Annual Report, 1903* (Atlanta, Georgia), n.p.

10. This photograph poses another important question: is the nurse a student or

a graduate? In this period, the staffs of many hospitals consisted primarily of students with few, if any, graduate nurses employed. This is, however, a generalization and does not hold true for all institutions. Therefore, unless I was able to determine the status of the nurse(s) in a photograph, the term nurse is used in its widest sense, encompassing both students and graduates.

11. "Rules and Regulations," *Luther Hospital and Training School* (Eau Claire, Wis.: Report dated 1905–1912), 26.

12. Ibid., 28.

13. L.R.G. Crandon and Albert Ehrenfried, *Surgical After-Treatment: A Manual of the Conduct of Surgical Convalescence,* 2d ed. (Philadelphia: W. B. Saunders, 1912), 29.

14. Ibid., 28.

15. Ibid., 31.

16. *Journal of the American Medical Association* 44 (10 June 1905): 1872.

17. Slide copies of the photographs reproduced in this essay and other historical nursing photographs are available from the Slide Archive of Historical Medical Photographs, State University of New York at Stony Brook, Health Sciences Library, P.O. Box 66, East Setauket, N.Y. 11733. See Apple, *Illustrated Catalogue.*

Karen Kingsley

3. The Architecture of Nursing*

Architecture has a role beyond that of providing space and shelter for human activities and institutions. Through its physical appearance—its forms and its ornamentation—architecture symbolizes the activity or the institution and tells us something about its importance within a culture. Nursing, when established as a profession in the nineteenth century, was as dependent as any other organization on architecture to establish its image to itself and to society.

In this study of the nurses' residence and the nurses' school, I will look at their origins and development in the late nineteenth century and then at their transformation in the twentieth century. I will discuss the architecture in terms of its physical response (for example, plan, spaces, etc.) to changing patterns in the living arrangements and education of nurses, as well as to shifts in general architectural styles. More important, I will investigate the way the built form reflects the social and cultural position of nursing. The focus of my inquiry is American residences and schools, but a brief discussion of the role of European prototypes and the ideas that inspired them is necessary to explain American developments.

There is no synthetic study on the architecture of nurses' residences and schools, although there is a large body of primary information. The data and ideas in this paper have been drawn from diverse sources including architectural journals, nursing and hospital journals, and historical records on individual nursing schools, as well as from discussions with nurses, hospital administrators, and architects. Each of these sources has its own particular approach to the topic and its own particular interest in it. But

*The information for this paper is drawn from many sources and articles. I particularly want to acknowledge nurses and hospital administrators at Charity Hospital School of Nursing and Tulane University Medical Center, New Orleans, and architects from Perez Associates, New Orleans, and Payette Associates, Boston. The principal journals consulted were *Modern Hospital, American Journal of Nursing, Hospitals, Architectural Forum, Architectural Record,* and *Pencil Points* (later *Progressive Architecture*).

from these sources, an argument can be developed about the architecture of nursing that illuminates the history and activity of nursing along with the way it was and is perceived in the culture at large.

Ideas and Intentions

The first Nightingale training school and nurses' "residence" opened at St. Thomas's Hospital in London in 1860 with fifteen students.[1] This school was such a revolutionary concept that it was planned as a two-year experimental program.[2] Although no special structure was built for the fifteen students, it is significant that a special living space was provided for them. The attic floor of one of the hospital blocks was converted for their "home." In writing about this first Nightingale school, Lucy Seymer notes that "to mould their characters, the probationers were required to live in a separate home under the supervision of a special sister."[3] Seymer states that the theory of nursing was taught in the wards in the form of clinical teaching, so it is doubtful any additional space was set aside to instruct the nurses in theory.[4] The larger part of the nurses' education—the practice—was, of course, conducted in the wards.

The nurses' "home" comprised a dining room, a sitting room, and separate sleeping compartments or cubicles for each pupil. These cubicles—each containing a bed, a chest of drawers, a washing stand, a chair, and a hanging press—did not provide complete privacy for each nurse; they were shaped by partitions that stopped six feet from the ceiling. But these quarters were found quite acceptable, as revealed in a probationer's letter describing the next temporary quarters—also an adaptive reuse—that the nurses occupied before a new residence was built:

> They brought me into a large, lofty, comfortable room, with tables, chairs, flowers, pictures, books, carpet, rug, fire, gas, like any sitting-room: off this, surrounded by the varnished boards, are the little bedroom cells, their wooden walls about ten feet high, not half way to the ceiling, with a bed, small chest of drawers, wash-stand, chair and towel-rail. The room was formerly a refreshment room, and is a very handsome and lofty one, lighted from the roof, and now surrounded by the nurses' cells, with the open space in the middle for their sitting-room, where I am now writing at one of the numerous little tables, with bright flowers and numbers of all kind of magazines around me. . . . I was taken to my room, provided with hot water, and after a little, called to tea, comfortably prepared in the nice light eating-room, quite separate from, but near our sitting-room . . . There is a temporary church fitted up in the house. . . .[5]

The architectural elements of the first Nightingale nursing residences and schools attempted to respond to a set of ideas about the profession of nursing as it was defined by Florence Nightingale. The Nightingale system of nursing consisted of three fundamental principles, all of which influenced the built form. First, Florence Nightingale insisted on "one female head" to have full power and responsibility over the nurses; she believed only a woman was capable of maintaining the discipline necessary for nursing. Thus, separate quarters for the superintendent or matron were provided within the house. Second, the students were to be trained in both the theory and the practice of nursing. Therefore, space for lectures and, later, demonstrations were included. Third, to ensure the character training essential for a good nurse, the students must live in "good accommodation" in a special home attached to the hospital. In approximately 1874, Florence Nightingale defined "good accommodation" or her ideal home and school as "A place of moral, religious and practical training; a place of training of character, habits, intelligence; a place to acquire knowledge, both technical and practical."[6] In 1892, she added:

> The first year of training in the Home is all-important—for it is there that order and discipline and method (of which possibly the probationers have had nothing as yet in their lives) must be first taught, or they will not be amenable to ward discipline.[7]

There was no detailed architectural program laid down by Nightingale, but she did formulate a set of ideas and principles about the training of nurses that influenced and shaped the physical form of the nurses' school and residence.

There were, though, two important architectural precedents historically associated with nursing: the monastery and the military hospital. The social organization of each was reflected architecturally in the individual cells or dormitory and the communal facilities for other activities. There is a clear relationship between the architectural components of these building types (especially the monastery) and the first residences: the dining room/refectory; the sitting room/parlor; the sleeping compartment/dormitory; the proximity but physical separation of the matron/abbess; and a small space set aside for intellectual endeavors. But monastic or military site-planning could not be followed at first because the Nightingale school was originally housed in temporary quarters. When St. Thomas's was rebuilt on a new site in 1871, the Nightingale home and school was located adjacent to the hospital, thus following Florence Nightingale's ideal. This building, designed by the architect according to Nightingale's guidelines for the training of nurses, provided single bedrooms for thirty-eight students. Separate quarters were incorporated for the matron. The architectural precedent was the physical organization of the monastery. A lecture room was provided in the basement.

In the United States, training school and hospital administrators followed English prototypes. They, too, considered it essential to provide comfortable and respectable accommodation in order to attract students from the social class—middle and with some education—they preferred. Previously, women who nursed had been perceived to have dubious morals, and the fledgling profession wanted to erase that image. As M. Adelaide Nutting, Superintendent of Nurses at the Johns Hopkins Hospital Training School from 1894 to 1907, wrote in 1898:

> We do not stand in the position of colleges and universities. . . . They do not vouch for character, but only for a certain degree of schooling. We stand in a different and peculiar position. We assume a moral responsibility for the character of the nurses we send out.[8]

Among its other achievements, the architecture helped establish the nurses' character in several ways.

The student nurses were predominantly young single women from small and medium-sized towns; it was as necessary to safeguard their character as to secure their safety.[9] The symbolic association of nursing with the monastic life, through the intermediary of architecture, reassured families that their daughters were in good hands. Certainly this association responded to broader social attitudes and pressures about unmarried women living apart from a family. This is a serious concern even today for hospitals and nursing school administrators in countries where women still lead restricted lives. Associations with the monastic ideal also must have helped put the nurses in the right frame of mind for a life of dedication and chastity.

The link between the new schools and nursing as a product of the monastery and military was reinforced further by the location of the residence. Whether housed in a part of the hospital building itself or in a separate building on the site of the hospital complex, the nurses were in close proximity to their work. This made eminently good sense for the hospital, since the long hours required of nurses in training and the exhausting nature of the work did not allow for commuting time or, as the nurses came to discover, for leisure activities.

The provision of a home, however, often placed a new financial burden on the hospital. In examining the history of the nursing residence and school, I found that cost consideration was frequently a major issue for both the hospital administration and the architect in their attempt to satisfy the nurses' training program within a very limited budget. As Lucy Seymer commented about plans for the first Nightingale school:

> It must be added that this insistence on a special "home" was subject to as much criticism as the rest of the system. Such a home may have been regarded by some as an unnecessary luxury; it also presented practical difficulties, since it added vastly to the expense of adopting the Nightingale plan. To employ these "new" nurses might mean for a hospital that a building had to be adapted for their use, or sometimes even specially built. This accommodation had to include not only bedrooms, but a sitting-room, and, perhaps also a dining-room, and rooms for the Home Sister. In the years that followed, when a group of nurses were sent from the School, the "triumvirate" were very particular about the quality and the suggested arrangement of the nurses' quarters.[10]

The criticism of luxury is a recurring theme in the history of nurses' residences.[11]

The Early Schools and Residences

A description of the nurses' accommodations at the Massachusetts General Hospital before the Boston Training School for Nurses opened in 1873 paints a terrible picture of the nurses' lives:

> The nurses slept in little rooms between the wards, two nurses occupying one bed, which was folded up during the day, and the room used for a sitting room, and frequently for a consulting room for the doctors, or for minor operations. One required to be on duty at 5 o'clock must, as can readily be imagined, make rather a hasty toilet. Consequently, the difficulties under which nurses labored, to keep themselves presentable in their little rooms, which were used as thoroughfares during the day, can hardly be exaggerated.[12]

But the nurses were not much better off in 1876 when, three years after the school had opened, they still did not have a residence and were lodged at several locations, including the attic of the main hospital building.

Makeshift and temporary quarters were a typical solution to the problem of housing students in the new schools of nursing founded in the late nineteenth century. The need and enthusiasm for trained nurses resulted in the establishment of schools before adequate living or teaching facilities were available or could be built. Just as the first Nightingale school at St. Thomas's Hospital in London was obliged to house its students in temporary spaces for its first eleven years, the first Nightingale school in the United States, at Bellevue Hospital, New York (it opened in 1873, a few months before the Boston Training School for Nurses), lodged its students in temporary quarters until a house was remodeled for the nurses in 1877.[13]

The small number of students in the early years of these schools and the fact that the nurses' training consisted mostly of ward practice made it feasible, if not always comfortable, to accommodate the students in converted or adapted existing space. But it soon became obvious to the schools that they could only expand and maintain their reputation, and influence and direct their nurses, when proper accommodations were provided. The Trustees of the Boston Training School for Nurses in their annual report of 1879 stated:

> We should be thankful to establish a nurses' home, where the nurses could live when not on duty. The Hospital accommodations are limited; they cannot give us a nurses' sitting room or separate bedroom, and our graduates are scattered the moment they leave the School. If we could provide a home, where the nurses serving in the Hospital could live when off duty; where the night watchers could have their daylight sleep under favorable circumstances, and to which our graduates could return in the intervals between their cases, we could better provide the most favorable conditions, and could more satisfactorily influence and control our nurses.[14]

Similarly, at the New York Hospital Training School, opened in 1877, the matron declared in 1879 that the accommodations were "too crowded" and "very unpleasant" and, moreover, that more privacy was needed to attract the right kind of student.[15] In that same year (1879), the school was given the temporary use of a house for sixty nurses. The annual report noted: "The founders of the School were impressed from the beginning with the importance of giving the nurses a home; not a mere lodging, but a comfortable home, where after their daily labors they may find relaxation and rest, free from the depressing influences of the Hospital," and added that "there is no doubt that the unusual exemption from illness which the nurses have enjoyed is largely owing to their cheerful and healthy surroundings. . . ."[16]

It was not until 1889 that the board of governors realized that a specially built home was needed to attract and retain pupils who were "women of refinement" and, therefore, absolutely necessary in order for the school to maintain its good reputation. The board also noted that the New York Hospital Training School was the only one at that time without a special home for the nurses.[17] Clearly, they felt at a disadvantage compared to other schools.

The idea that there should be a special and separate building that would contain comfortable residential space—that there should be a physical entity devoted solely to the needs of nurses—was firmly established by the late nineteenth century. Several reasons motivated this idea, although the degree of importance of any or all of the reasons varied from school to school.

Before anything, it was essential to attract the right kind of student to the school. The Board of Managers of the Pennsylvania Hospital Training School for Nurses, founded in 1876, expressed this goal when it agreed that "educated women" would be "productive of good to the hospital."[18] Pleasant surroundings and favorable conditions would attract a better class of student, and that would benefit the hospital.

The smooth running of the hospital could only be assured, as well, through the physical and mental well-being of the nurses, through their being comfortable and happy in their lodging: cheerful and healthy surroundings made contented nurses. If care were given the nurses, it would be reflected in the quantity and quality of care given by the nurses to the patients. A. C. Hutchinson outlined in a letter the reasons for his donation for the construction of a residence for the nurses of Charity Hospital in New Orleans in 1901. He was convinced that the nurses must live comfortably for the good of the patient and, by extension, the good of the hospital.[19]

Once the student was accepted into the school, hospital administrators preferred to provide a single bedroom for each student because they believed the kind of women they wanted had no experience of sharing.[20] Administrators were also concerned that shared rooms might prove disruptive to the smooth running of the school by mixing social classes. Single rooms made it easier to influence and control the nurses, a major concern with administrators. The architecture of the residence was as important an element as any in the development of the training program. The residence provided more than shelter. It controlled the nurse's physical activity and social interactions and, thus, truly molded her character and attitudes.

Almost all the goals and problems encountered and confronted by the first schools of nursing in the late nineteenth century are present in the early years of the Johns Hopkins Hospital Training School.[21] The student nurses at the Johns Hopkins Hospital Training School spent less time than most in temporary quarters, for a training school was planned as an integral part of the hospital founded by Johns Hopkins in 1873 and opened in 1885. The nurses' home and training school, opened in 1889, was located on the periphery of the hospital site (Fig. 3-1). Considered far superior to any residence built so far, it had accommodations for fifty nurses, a lecture room, a training kitchen, and reception rooms. It was described as resembling a "first-class hotel" and was designed to create an atmosphere in contrast to that of the nurses' work place.[22] But increasing student enrollment saw two students to a single room before five years had passed. The expansion of the original two-year training program to three years, in 1896, soon made additional accommodation even more imperative. Students were initially lodged over the pharmacy; then, in 1904, one of the private wards was taken over. But as with other schools, this satisfied only the need for sleeping accommodations; there was no corresponding growth in classrooms. Finally, in 1907, two wings were added to the original nurses' home, and all the students were together once more.

Of great importance for the profession, the provision of a new and separate building made dramatically clear the difference between "old" nursing and "new" nursing, of the untrained nurse from the trained nurse. Unceremoniously lodged together, nurses could not have felt any level of prestige attributed to their work. As has been shown at Massachusetts General Hospital, before the first schools were established, nurses were housed in worse conditions than most servants. An imagery of prestige, recognizable to the public, was essential if nurses were to achieve the recognition necessary for the new profession. A separate and substantial building with a distinctive architectural character devoted to the nurses' studies and private lives proclaimed a new image.

The nurses' residence and school presented to architects and to their clients the challenge of designing a completely new building type. The size of the building and the internal organization of space were determined by the requirements of the program: numbers and size of bedrooms, sitting room, dining room, lecture room, and, perhaps, demonstration rooms, and kitchens. The interior of the building—its degree of individual space for the nurses, its furnishings and fittings—gave to the nurses their necessary comfort and their self-image. Architects provided

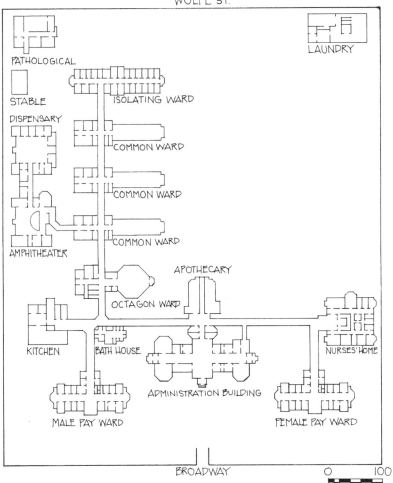

WOLFE ST.

PATHOLOGICAL

LAUNDRY

STABLE

ISOLATING WARD

DISPENSARY

COMMON WARD

COMMON WARD

COMMON WARD

AMPHITHEATER

APOTHECARY

OCTAGON WARD

KITCHEN

BATH HOUSE

NURSES' HOME

ADMINISTRATION BUILDING

MALE PAY WARD

FEMALE PAY WARD

BROADWAY

0   100

FIGURE 3-1. Johns Hopkins Hospital Training School, Baltimore. Site plan as
built, 1885. From John S. Billings, *Description of the Johns Hopkins Hospital* (Baltimore: Johns Hopkins Hospital, 1890), pl. 2. Reprinted in John D. Thompson
and Grace Goldin, *The Hospital: A Social and Architectural History* (New Haven:
Yale University Press, 1975), 185, fig. 184. Copyright © 1975 by Yale University.
Published with permission of Yale University Press. Redrawn by Daniel Shirk.

most of these interiors with spacious living rooms and single bedrooms to help administrators attract, retain, and mold the nurses.

But it was the exterior of the building that would establish the image of the nurse and the nursing profession to the broader public; the presence of the nursing school and residence was a constant and tangible indicator and reminder. It is commonplace in the history of architecture that new social and political institutions or new rulers reinforce their identity and power through the medium of architecture; it was and is a commonly understood symbol.[23] Of all the elements that gave status to the nursing profession—and this status frequently met resistance by doctors and administrators in the early years—the building dedicated solely to this profession was an important indicator of its arrival and stature in society.

But this new typology had to be designed to present an appearance that was appropriate to its function and purpose. Late nineteenth-century architecture is distinguished by its eclecticism, drawing at will on any historical precedent deemed fit. The Boston Training School for Nurses followed the then fashionable Renaissance palace or Italianate style. Similarly, the residence for the nurses (separate from the Sisters' home) built in 1901 for Charity Hospital School of Nursing in New Orleans, like the nurses' residence at Johns Hopkins Hospital Training School, adopted a rather austere Renaissance form (Fig. 3-2). The smooth wall surfaces, the order and symmetry of the forms and details, all defined by a strong cornice, found favor with the architects of nurses' schools. Moreover, the Renaissance palace was particularly appropriate, for it is, historically, the archetypal urban residence. The plainness and decorum of the type, compared to other more richly ornamented structures, made it a suitable style for its new function. It was a style that could assure the public that the building—and thus the nurses—were clean, that there were no nooks, crevices, or protuberances for germs to lodge in and multiply.[24]

Not all the architects of these early schools of nursing, though, chose to go Neo-Renaissance. The residence for the Training School for Nurses of the Hospital of the University of Pennsylvania, constructed in 1886, was closer to the typically American suburban domestic ideal (Fig. 3-3). A two-story building of brick with stone trim and covered by a steep, pitched roof, it spoke of respectability and stability. It included a library and parlor along with the single bedrooms for twenty-six nurses. No recreational facilities were provided.

Simple forms and designs, modesty, no emotional abundance of applied columns and pilasters, no rich extravaganza of sculpture, no fripperies or

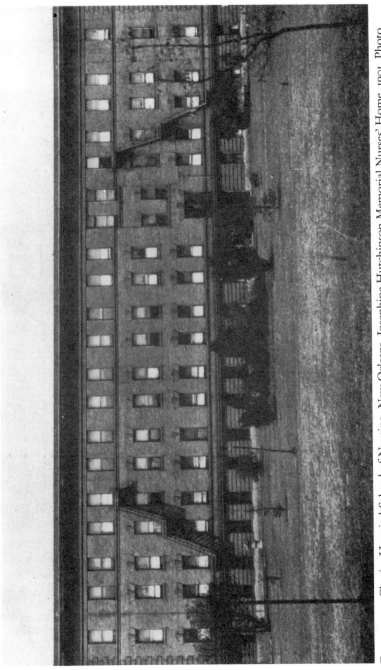

FIGURE 3-2. Charity Hospital School of Nursing, New Orleans. Josephine Hutchinson Memorial Nurses' Home, 1901. Photo courtesy Charity Hospital School of Nursing.

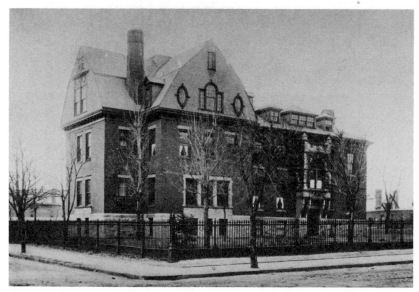

FIGURE 3-3. Training School for Nurses of the Hospital of the University of Pennsylvania, Philadelphia. Wood Memorial Nurses' Home, 1886. Photo courtesy Hospital of the University of Pennsylvania.

frivolities—these were not solely a matter of budget considerations. They were as much the need to proclaim the serious nature and purpose of this new institution of nursing. The nurses' residence and school had to speak of the skill, rigor, discipline, efficiency, and respectability of its inhabitants.

The Renaissance palace form adopted at Boston and Charity, and at many other schools, was perceived in the late nineteenth century as especially suitable for public and educational monuments, particularly if they were in urban locations, as were most early nursing schools. That style possessed enough of a domestic image to be appropriate for a women's establishment, but it was not the particular style that mattered as much as that the building be "in style." The *presence* of architectural style was what counted. With the monumental and fashionable independent building, the nursing profession could publicly declare its identity and importance in society.

The training school was usually a free-standing building and invariably located on the periphery of the hospital grounds. This gave the nurses a group identity separate from, but belonging to, a larger unit. The physical nature of her world taught the student nurse that she had no life beyond her residence and the hospital—and it taught the public that her life was intimately tied to the hospital, and, therefore, to their welfare. She was the institution and the institution was she: she breathed, ate, and slept hospital. The nurse's life was completely regulated by strict rules for rising, eating, studying, and working. Subsumed into a world that could and should provide all her needs and desires, she was required by that world, in turn, to give her all, physically and spiritually. The nursing profession held a double-edged sword. It offered for the young woman in the late nineteenth century the opportunity of a profession, an alternative to marriage, and freedom from the restraints of the house and societal mores. But it also cloistered its pupils and instilled in them the same values—of loyalty and self-sacrifice—and physically separated them from a broader social milieu. Nursing, in its evolution from the cloister and the military, adopted similar architectural concepts and forms to satisfy its ideological needs: self-sufficient communities in the service of a goal that denied individual self-sufficiency.

Into the Twentieth Century

Increasing numbers of student nurses outstripping facilities continued to be a problem in the first decades of the twentieth century. Expansion of the training course from two years to three at many schools and a slightly shortened work week—to, for example, fifty-four hours per week at Bellevue by 1920—exacerbated the difficulties. Frequently, the only solution was to house two students in a room designed for one until better facilities could be provided. But since the success of a hospital depended in large part on the health and welfare of its student nurses, administrators felt increasing pressure to ensure that the student was loyal, content, and hardworking despite the long hours. One solution was to make the nurses feel as if they were part of a caring and loving community, a sort of extended family. Nurses were encouraged to see their residence as a real "home," and the emphasis on the homelike attributes of the residence became one of the primary architectural considerations. As early as 1896, the managers of the University of Pennsylvania School had expressed concern about the ambience of the residence:

> The life of a nurse is necessarily an exacting and fatiguing one. She should when off duty be able to retire to convenient, cheerful, and well-appointed rooms, with facilities for bathing and personal hygiene. Nothing is more calculated to secure the best class of women for this important work than comfortable home-like surroundings.[25]

A residence that was more than merely pleasant, that had the attributes of home life, came to be perceived as central to good nursing morale. A family spirit in the nurses was seen as the key to creating a family atmosphere in the hospital. The latter would help attract and retain patients. If architecture had played its most important roles as a means of ordering and forming the character of the nurses and as a symbolic statement of the profession in the late nineteenth century, the twentieth century was to put new demands on it. It now had to satisfy the social and familial needs of the nurses.

After World War I, labor turnover in the nursing profession became an increasing problem. By 1923, the Report of the Committee for the Study of Nursing Education openly acknowledged that better living conditions were a crucial means of attracting and keeping students of good caliber. The committee recognized that societal mores had changed to the extent that it was no longer possible to invoke monastic or militaristic ideals, that it was necessary, instead, to get the cooperation of the nurses rather than to enforce discipline.[26]

The committee recommended that the nurse should upon entering her "home" after work step into a different atmosphere. In architectural terms, it specified that the living quarters be detached from the hospital buildings and out of range of the work place. A single bedroom for each student nurse was seen as the ideal because it gave the student a place to get away from people. (More than half the schools at this time had double rooms and some housed up to ten students in a dormitory room.) Recognizing that the students worked long hours and had little time or energy for social life, the committee felt that social needs were best provided in the residence.

Provisions for recreation had been incorporated as early as 1912 at the Boston Training School, where a gymnasium had been included in the additions to its residence, and in other schools students were permitted to use a college swimming pool. Most of the new schools built in the 1920s and after followed the committee's recommendations and included a gymnasium and swimming pool, as well as nearby tennis courts, as a matter of course. In terms of the homelike qualities of the new residences, there were a number of options, each, though, dependent on the amount of site space, climate, and budget. If an outside sitting area—a patio or terrace—could not be provided, as was the case with many urban schools, a roof-garden was. Additional comforts or conveniences included, where climate permitted, outside sleeping porches opening from the bedrooms and sit-

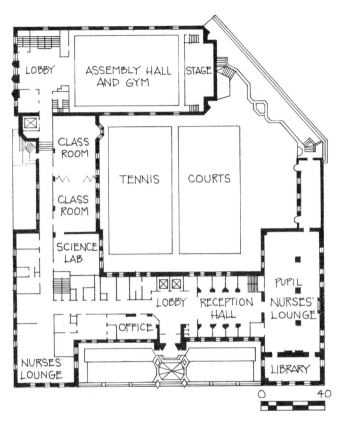

FIGURE 3-4. St. Francis General Hospital School of Nursing, Pittsburgh. First-floor plan of building, also showing tennis courts from ground floor below, 1929–31. From *Modern Hospital* 34 (March 1930): 92–93. Redrawn by Daniel Shirk. (The redrawing combines two drawings, which contain plans of two different floors, into one drawing.)

ting rooms on each floor. Sitting rooms were also designed large enough for social events such as informal dances.

The twelve-story nurses' home at St. Francis General Hospital School of Nursing in Pittsburgh was typical (Fig. 3-4).[27] Built between 1929 and 1931, it incorporated a swimming pool, a gymnasium equipped with a stage for events, a bowling alley, reception and tea rooms, lounges, and a sun room. The first floor contained classrooms, science laboratories, and a library. Individual rooms were provided for the four hundred nurses, and these were designed to be large enough for the necessary furniture but small enough to prevent their being used for two beds. Each bedroom measured fourteen feet by eight feet and was eight-and-a-half feet high. The home was organized around a courtyard in which the tennis courts were located. The plan is strongly reminiscent of monastic layouts. Moreover, although the number and kinds of activities for the nurses grew, the physical location of them did not. The cloistered life prevailed.

Elaboration or "decoration" of the interior of the home became an increasingly standard means of deinstitutionalizing the residence and of enriching the nurses' home life. The choices of furniture, of curtains, and of color were important issues in both the hospital and architectural journals. But from residence to residence, the size of the room varied little and the furniture of each—built-in desks, bookcases, and closets—was as uniform. Of the many residences featured in the journals of the 1920s and 1930s (and especially in *Modern Hospital*) emphasis was placed on the living areas— parlors, sitting rooms, lobbies—and little attention paid to the educational facilities.

One area of the building that always received special attention by both architect and journal was the entrance. As one observer commented about nursing residences in general: "While plain details of finish make the care of the home less irksome, there should be enough detail to give interest; the entrance, at least should possess some architectural merit."[28] A specially designed entrance and lobby, different from those of nearby buildings, provided monumentality and, by extension, gave the nurses identity and stature. The magnificent doors of the St. Francis General Hospital School of Nursing graphically depict the nurses' world; the panels are individually designed to show the tools of the trade—microscopes, beds, stethoscopes, and so on (Fig. 3-5). The elaborate or grand entrance, as it is intended to, also made leaving and arriving a special event in the daily round of the nurse (Figs. 3-6, 3-7). As a place of transition or passage from one activity to another, it emphasized the separation between work and home.[29]

In urban areas where no distant and complete view of the building could be provided, architects had to find additional means to monumentalize and individualize the residence and school. A frequent recourse was the elaboration of the top of the building. The Lincoln School for Nurses in New York, besides its magnificent angled entrance, was enriched by a pseudoclassical temple at the summit of its eight stories (Fig. 3-7). As well as giving the building prominence in a dense urban setting, the temple had the added value of referring to ideal classical civilizations.[30]

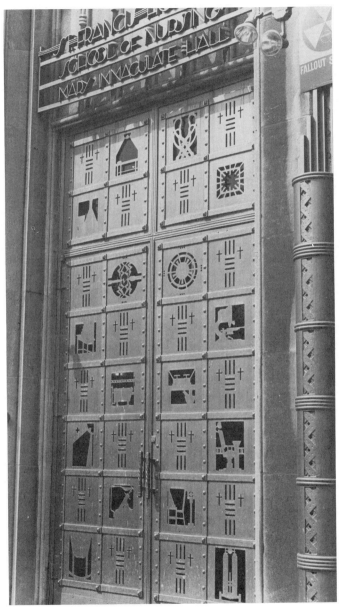

FIGURE 3-5. St. Francis General Hospital School of Nursing, Pittsburgh. Entrance Doors, 1929–31. Photo courtesy St. Francis General Hospital.

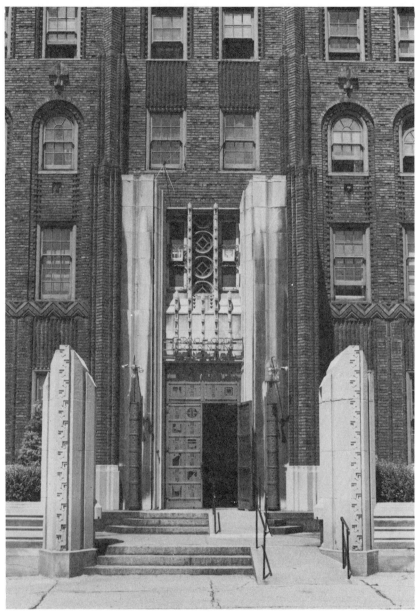

FIGURE 3-6. St. Francis General Hospital School of Nursing, Pittsburgh. Entrance, 1929–31. Photo courtesy St. Francis General Hospital.

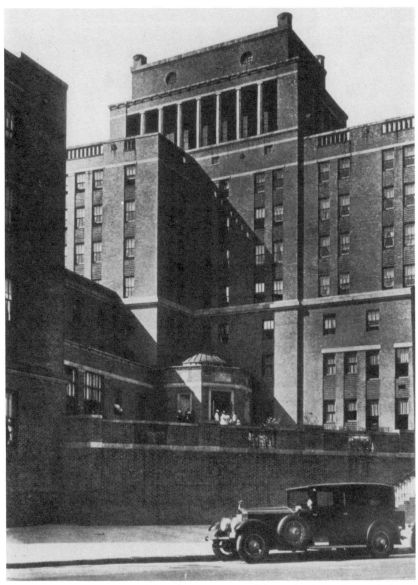

FIGURE 3-7. Lincoln School for Nurses, New York. Exterior, 1929. From *Architectural Forum* 51 (October 1929): 499, pl. 118. Photo by S. H. Gottscho. Reprinted with permission of Watson-Guptill Publications, Inc.

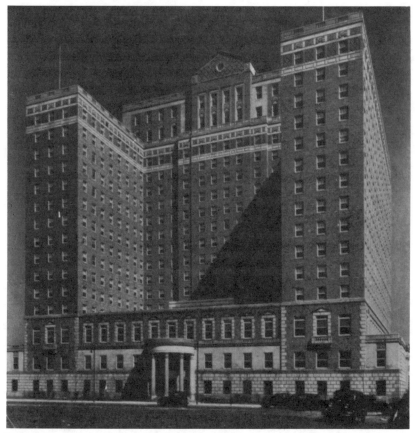

FIGURE 3-8. Cook County Hospital Nurses' Home, Chicago. Exterior, 1935.
From *Public Buildings: A Survey of Architecture* (Washington, D.C.: U.S. Government Printing Office, 1939), 372.

Nurses' residences were likened by both critics and architects to hotels, and the comparison was not inappropriate. For the architect, the programmatic requirements for an urban nurses' residence and school were similar to those of a hotel: a multistory building that could sleep a large number of people. Accordingly, their design was similar to that of a hotel. To provide light to all the rooms, architects generally planned a U, H, or E shape, an architectural organization that provided interior courtyards or wells of light. With the expansion of hospital care and the increased need for nurses, the newly constructed residence and school combinations were often very large. For example, the nurses' home of Cook County Hospital in Chicago, completed in 1935, occupied an entire city block (Fig. 3-8). H-

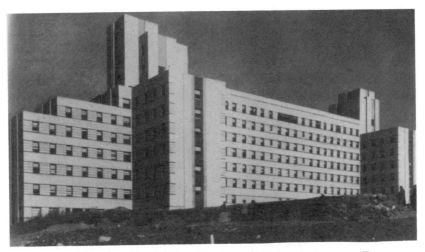

FIGURE 3-9. Nurses' Home, Welfare Island, New York. Exterior, 1937. From *Public Buildings: A Survey of Architecture* (Washington, D.C.: U.S. Government Printing Office, 1939), 345.

shaped in plan, it was seventeen stories tall. Lecture rooms and demonstration, anatomy, and chemistry laboratories were located on the ground floor. The first and second floors contained separate dining rooms and lounges for graduate and student nurses, administration offices, more lecture rooms, and a library. Above these floors were 817 bedrooms for nurses.[31]

But nurses' residences, like all medical facilities, were distinguishable from hotels in the 1920s and 1930s: they were much plainer. They were the ideal architectural typology for architects of that rational and progressive age, and by the late 1930s they had adopted the look of progressive modernity in a clean, efficient, and functional appearance that symbolized the time. The nurses' home on Welfare Island in the East River, New York, completed in 1937, was typical of later 1930s hospital design (Fig. 3-9). Almost as large—with six hundred single bedrooms—as the nurses' home of Cook County Hospital, it had the same separation of educational spaces from sleeping spaces.[32]

The decoration of the nurses' residence in the first decades of the twentieth century was more luxurious than before, and opportunities for recreation were increased, but in one major way nineteenth-century ideas prevailed: that the academic part of the training program take place in the residence. Since this element of the curriculum had expanded considerably by the 1920s, a much larger area of the residence had to be given over to classrooms and demonstration rooms. Whenever possible, all the teaching spaces were clustered and on a single floor or adjacent floors and preferably at ground level. The upper floors served as home.

The building, then, served both as a home—with the idea of escape from work—and as classroom, which denied the logic of the first. In an ambiguous situation at best, the student nurse could escape work only by removing herself even further from the "real" world by retreating upward in the building into the privacy or isolation of her bedroom. Principally, though, the nurses' home and school was seen as a residence rather than as a place of education. Most of the building was devoted to bedrooms, and the public image of the nurse was, therefore, of someone who lived in a dormitory and learned her profession in the hospital.

Since World War II

The severe shortage of nurses after World War II provided the impetus for federal funding to improve existing facilities and construct new ones. In 1957, hospitals were brought within the College Housing Program, thus making them eligible for forty-year, low-interest loans for the provision of student housing. This resulted in a great burst of building activity; within five years, sixty hospitals with nursing schools had residences finished or in progress.[33] Then, the Nurse Training Act of 1964 provided ninety million dollars of funding for construction and expansion of nursing education facilities.[34]

Hospital administrators were perfectly aware that the nursing situation determined the whole hospital operation.[35] To attract students, they increasingly emphasized the physical amenities offered the potential student nurse. It had been demonstrated that investment in physical facilities made good economic sense. Buildings last a long time and with all their recreational and social facilities had tangible appeal for a young woman trying to decide on a career. Moreover, the residence—as opposed to the wages paid to the nurses- -was often funded by a source other than the hospital. Thus, further efforts to deinstitutionalize the residence were made; the hotel or the women's club was the ideal to emulate.

A major change in the education of the nurse occurred in the 1960s. Education was no longer conceived as an arm of service to the hospital. With this revolution in the concept of what nursing education meant, the architecture of nursing changed. Until then, the joint residence and school was a dormitory, not an education building; little space was given over to

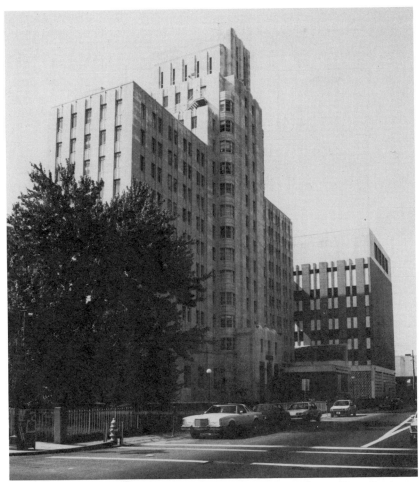

FIGURE 3-10. Charity Hospital School of Nursing, New Orleans. Sister Stanislaus Memorial Home and Education Building. Exterior, 1939 and 1973. Photo by and courtesy of Daniel Shirk.

education.[36] By the 1960s, rather than bundle training and residence into one architectural package, it was seen as preferable to separate work space from living areas whenever possible.

On the university campus, as just one of many buildings, the nurses' school became anonymous. In urban centers, new nurses' schools were indistinguishable from office buildings. The education wing of Charity Hospital School of Nursing illustrates the point (Fig. 3-10).[37] Yet much remains traditional in the design of new facilities. The Bechtel School of

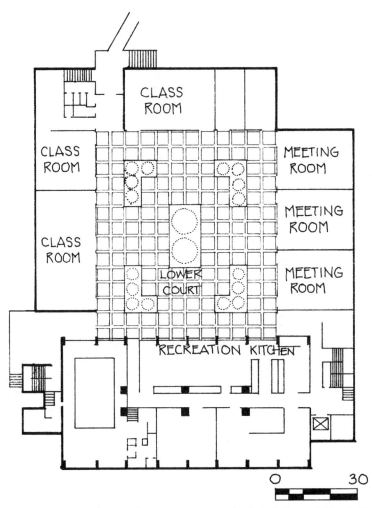

FIGURE 3-11. Bechtel School of Nursing (now Bechtel Hall, Samuel Merrit Hospital College of Nursing) and Residence, Oakland. Plan, 1966, by the architects, Stone, Marracini and Patterson. From *Architectural Record* 141 (May 1967): 163. Published with permission of *Architectural Record*. Redrawn by Daniel Shirk.

Nursing (now College of Nursing) and Residence of Samuel Merritt Hospital, Oakland, follows the pattern of the school and residence in one building (Fig. 3-11). Organized around an interior court, it continues to refer to the monastery cloister. The lower two floors of the seven-story building contain classrooms, study rooms, and recreation areas, and the upper floors consist of bedrooms. The bedrooms were designed as double rooms, not single.[38]

Whether two buildings or one, the ideal of well-crafted and spacious buildings came up against the reality of costs. For administrators to stay within limited budgets, students were increasingly lodged two to a room. This had been a solution in and from the financially depressed 1930s and evidently an unwelcome one judging from the creative ways such cost cutting was justified by hospital administrators. Sharing was described as democratic or as a local tradition for students unfamiliar with a room of one's own.[39] The reduction of personal living space was considered far more acceptable to school administrators than the abandonment of enticements such as swimming pools, gymnasiums, and lounges.

It is interesting to examine one of the major new nursing facilities built recently. The School of Nursing of the Aga Khan University in Karachi, Pakistan, designed in 1972, opened in February 1981. Part of a teaching hospital complex, the school is located on the periphery of the site (Figs. 3-12, 3-13). The buildings organized around courtyards respond to traditional regional architecture as well as to a scheme suitable for nurses' residences and schools. The school is sumptuous, made possible by a large budget and the Aga Khan's interest in reviving traditional Islamic crafts and ornament (Figs. 3-14, 3-15). But the program called for a lavish building to establish a set of ideas about nursing. Nurses in Pakistan previously suffered low status and were poorly paid and housed. In addition, many students are from strict Muslim families and the school has to provide the assurance that the young women will be safe and well cared for. As the architects stated: "These assurances are symbolized by the architecture."[40] As with so many schools of nursing, this one, too, has received criticism that the luxuries will spoil the nurses, making them unfit to deal with real life. The architects claim, however, that it is precisely such luxuries, rather than merely the provision of basic amenities, that speak of the value of the nurse in society. The Aga Khan School is the history of the architecture of nursing repeating itself. In those areas of the world where nursing is still a new profession for women, architectural solutions repeat those made in nineteenth-century England and America.

Conclusion

Architecture is the principal expression of how people live—physically, socially, intellectually, and spiritually; it touches on all aspects of peoples' lives and values. To express the image of the nurse, the architecture of nursing had to satisfy a number of demands. Perhaps the most important

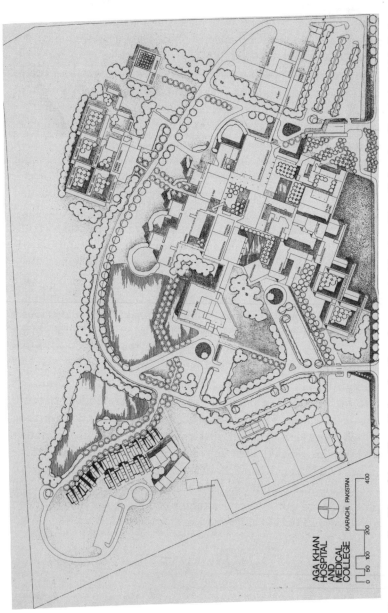

FIGURE 3-12. Site Plan of Aga Khan University Complex, 1972–81. The Aga Khan University, Hospital and Medical College, Karachi, Pakistan. Architects: Payette Associates. Design Consultant: Mozhan Khadem. Photo courtesy Payette Associates and The Aga Khan University Hospital, Karachi.

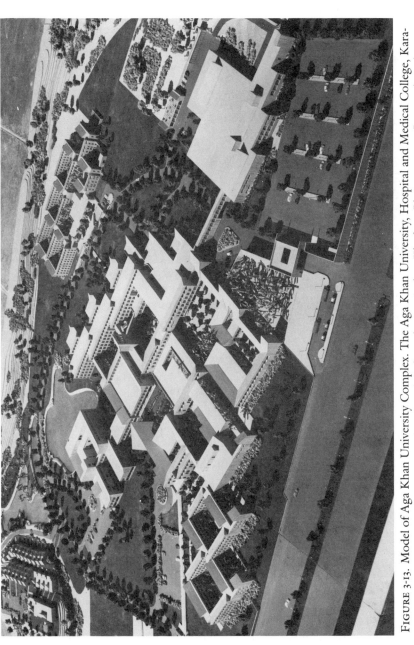

FIGURE 3-13. Model of Aga Khan University Complex. The Aga Khan University, Hospital and Medical College, Karachi, Pakistan. Architects: Payette Associates. Design Consultant: Mozhan Khadem. Photo courtesy Payette Associates and The Aga Khan University Hospital, Karachi.

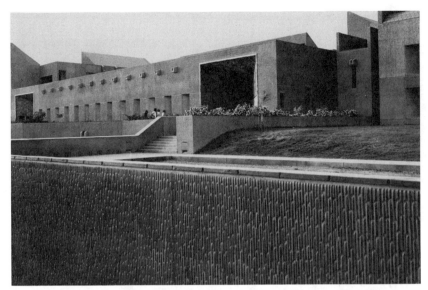

FIGURE 3-14. View of Entrance and Surrounding Wall. The Aga Khan University, Hospital and Medical College, Karachi, Pakistan. Architects: Payette Associates. Design Consultant: Mozhan Khadem. Photo courtesy Payette Associates and The Aga Khan University Hospital, Karachi.

in the early years of the profession was to give nursing an identity and a status. The monumental, independent building devoted solely to that profession established its worth to society. This stature was enhanced by the building's being of a fashionable style, although sufficiently domestic in appearance and demure in regard to ornamentation to establish the caring and serious nature of the nurses' character and work. The architecture had to erase the old image of the nurse from the mind of the public and establish a new one.

At the same time that the architecture declared the existence of the new trained nurses, it also was used to recruit into that profession. Instead of shorter hours or more pay, it was economically more feasible in the long run for hospitals to provide more luxurious accommodation and facilities for the nurses. So, the idea of *a* building, that is, its separateness or pure existence as being sufficient, as was true during the establishment of the profession in the late nineteenth century, became insufficient to attract students in the twentieth century. The contents of the building—swimming pool, gymnasium, reception rooms—increasingly came to be stressed. It also had to provide the qualities of a home away from home.

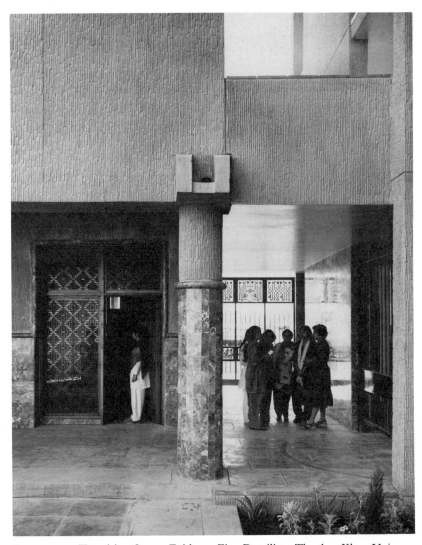

FIGURE 3-15. Transition Spaces Evidence Fine Detailing. The Aga Khan University, Hospital and Medical College, Karachi, Pakistan. Architects: Payette Associates. Design Consultant: Mozhan Khadem. Photo courtesy Payette Associates and The Aga Khan University Hospital, Karachi.

The architecture of nursing from its inception until very recently was principally residential. It did not and could not alter until a changed concept of the education of the nurse occurred and the curriculum shifted its emphasis from practice to theory. From that time, teaching space—the school—became an important architectural entity in itself. Once the two buildings were physically separated, the nurse could be seen as independent from the dormitory and, ultimately, the cloister or the military, and no longer perceived as a mere handmaiden of the hospital. Yet, at the same time, the relentless anonymity of the new buildings of the 1960s diminished a sense of identity many nurses had with their school and hospital.

The architecture of nursing, by its public physical presence, established the image of the nurse long before most people had experience with her. The architecture was a fundamental means of making socially acceptable the new and radical institution of nursing. What the architecture had to state about the nurse told potential patients, too, about the hospital: that it was up-to-date, safe and sober, and, through disciplined, virtuous, and sisterly nurses, would carefully shelter and restore the sick to health.

Notes

1. See Lucy Seymer, *Florence Nightingale's Nurses: The Nightingale Training School, 1860–1960* (London: Pitman Medical Publishing Company, 1960), for a general discussion of the physical arrangements of the temporary residences.
2. Lucy Ridgely Seymer, "One Hundred Years Ago . . . ," *American Journal of Nursing* 60 (May 1960): 659.
3. Ibid.
4. Ibid., 661.
5. Letter from one probationer (Agnes Jones) to her family, quoted in Seymer, *Florence Nightingale's Nurses*, 29.
6. Quoted in Seymer, *Florence Nightingale's Nurses*, 35.
7. Ibid. The importance of order and discipline in the training of American nurses was expressed by Lavinia Dock, Assistant Superintendent at Johns Hopkins Hospital Training School in 1893: "The organization of a school is and must be military"; see Jane E. Mottus, *New York Nightingales: The Emergence of the Nursing Profession at Bellevue and New York Hospital, 1850–1920* (Ann Arbor: UMI Research Press, 1981), 185.
8. Quoted in Nancy Tomes, "'Little World of Our Own': The Pennsylvania Hospital Training School for Nurses, 1895–1907," *Journal of the History of Medicine and Allied Sciences* 33 (October 1978): 515.
9. Ibid., 518. Tomes has assembled statistics on the backgrounds of student nurses for the Pennsylvania Hospital Training School. They are confirmed by

other schools: see, for example, Mottus, 49 and 59; and Seymer, *Florence Nightingale's Nurses,* 17.

10. Seymer, *Florence Nightingale's Nurses,* 35.

11. See, for example, Sister M. Laurentine, "A Nurses' Home That Promises to Be a Home in Its Truest Sense," *Modern Hospital* 34 (March 1930): 92.

12. Quoted in Sara E. Parsons, *History of the Massachusetts General Hospital Training School for Nurses* (Boston: Whitcomb & Barrows, 1922), 6.

13. For Bellevue, see Mottus, 49, 54–55, and 70.

14. Quoted in Parsons, 49.

15. Mottus, 80.

16. Quoted in Parsons, 49.

17. Mottus, 82.

18. Quoted in Tomes, 509.

19. The letter is in the Archives in the Library of the Charity Hospital School of Nursing, New Orleans.

20. Tomes, 522; see also Parsons, 49.

21. For Johns Hopkins, see Ethel Johns and Blanche Pfefferkorn, *The Johns Hopkins School of Nursing, 1889–1949* (Baltimore: Johns Hopkins Press, 1954); "Progress in the Hospital," *Johns Hopkins Nurses Alumnae Magazine* 7 (March 1908): 5–12; and Patience Carr, "Hampton House," *Johns Hopkins Nurses Alumnae Magazine* 25 (November 1926): 203–7.

22. Johns and Pfefferkorn, 21–22.

23. The artistic assertion of "arrival" is a recognized historical phenomenon. It begins with the transformation of a building type to serve new needs, for example, the secular Roman basilica taken over and adopted for the Christian Church. For an excellent discussion of the use of architecture as a political and social statement, see Oleg Grabar, "The Symbolic Appropriation of the Land," in *The Formation of Islamic Art* (New Haven: Yale University Press, 1973), 45–74.

24. For illustrations of Boston, see Parsons, 57; for Johns Hopkins, see *Johns Hopkins Nurses Alumnae Magazine* 7 (March 1908): 2.

25. Quoted in Mary Virginia Stephenson, *The First Fifty Years of the Training School for Nurses of the Hospital of the University of Pennsylvania* (Philadelphia: J. B. Lippincott, 1940), 73. The importance of the homelike qualities of the residence can be seen just in the titles of articles on nurses' residences published in, for example, *Modern Hospital* during the 1920s and 1930s. Two examples are Paul Gerhardt, Jr., "A Nurses' Home Planned to Ensure a Contented Personnel" 35 (September 1930): 83–86; and Edward Randall and Lucius R. Wilson, "Nurses Should Be Happy in This Well Planned Home," 40 (March 1933): 69–74. See also my notes 11 and 31 for additional titles.

26. *Nursing and Nursing Education in the United States, Report of the Committee for the Study of Nursing Education* (New York: Macmillan, 1923), 442–53. See also Lavinia Dock's similar opinion, changed from her earlier views (my note 7) in Lavinia L. Dock and Isabel M. Stewart, *A Short History of Nursing* (New York: Putnam, 1925), 381.

27. Laurentine, 92–93.

28. Edward F. Stevens, "The Nurses' Residence," *Modern Hospital* 18 (April 1922): 323.

29. It is ironic that these entrances were not to be enjoyed by the student nurses on a day-to-day basis. Shirley Steele, Professor in the School of Nursing of the University of Alabama in Birmingham, informs me that the main entrance at some schools was for guests and special events. Nurses had a side entrance.

30. "Lincoln School for Nurses," *Architectural Forum* 51 (October 1929): 499–503.

31. Margaret R. Griffin, "Nurses at Cook County Have a Homelike Home," *Modern Hospital* 46 (February 1936): 70–74; and C. W. Short and R. Stanley-Brown, *Public Buildings* (Washington, D.C.: U.S. Government Printing Office, 1939), 372.

32. Short and Stanley-Brown, 345.

33. Jay Du Von, "Federal Loan Program Stimulates Student Housing Construction," *Hospitals* (Journal of the American Hospital Association) 36 (1 April 1962): 49.

34. "Nursing Education Facilities," *Architectural Record* 141 (May 1967): 159.

35. "Nurses Home Attracts Vital Personnel," *Architectural Record* 115 (March 1954): 172.

36. Discussion (5 July 1983) with Sister Blanche MacDonnell, Director of Education of Charity Hospital, New Orleans, and formerly Director of the School of Nursing at Charity Hospital.

37. The school and residence of Charity Hospital School of Nursing was converted into a residence only, and a new education building was attached. The original school is visually unified with Charity Hospital (all built in the late 1930s) and, typically, is located on the edge of the hospital complex site. The new education wing, finished in 1973, completely disregards its architectural context. The new wing is, though, handsomely equipped with swimming pool, gymnasium, library, visual aids department, laboratories, etc.

38. "Nursing Education Facilities," 163.

39. For democracy, see W. M. Breitinger, "A Nurses' Home That Combines Luxury, Space, Comfort," *Modern Hospital* 36 (April 1931): 66; for local tradition, see Charles H. McCauley, "Nurses' Home, Memorial Hospital, Anniston, Alabama," *Progressive Architecture* 28 (November 1947): 80.

40. Mildred F. Schmertz, "Setting a Standard for Architecture in Islam: The Aga Khan School of Nursing in Karachi Designed by Payette Associates and Mozhan Khadem," *Architectural Record* 169 (October 1981): 84.

Part II

Images in Literature

The four essays in Part II consider images of nurses and nursing in literature and are arranged in roughly chronological order, according to the literature they discuss. The first essay goes back to ancient myths and archetypes to find sources of negative modern images of nurses. The second essay seeks positive literary images of nurses and finds them in nineteenth- and twentieth-century characterizations of men who care for the sick and wounded. The third essay analyzes nurse characters depicted in selected twentieth-century short stories. And the fourth essay analyzes the three nurse characters in a recent novel by a Nobel prize–winning author. The first and third essays include some popular works; the second and fourth deal only with mainstream literature.

These literary essays, then, remind us of the gap between high culture and popular culture, between what used to be called highbrow and low-brow culture. The "canon," that body of highbrow works selected to be perpetuated by being taught to college students, has traditionally excluded the work of women and ethnic minorities. For centuries in Western culture, men have been the patrons of the arts, as well as the artists and writers. Thus, the cultural images that reign in the canon are, for the most part, created by men, for men. Because the canon is so systematically taught, it shapes the common cultural expectations and attitudes of the educated class. Women, as well as men, internalize its images and values.

Implicit in this question of high versus popular culture is the related issue of class. Traditionally men were better educated than women; thus, male physicians were (historically, anyway) more likely than female nurses to have studied the canon. The implications of this educational (and class) difference are worth some speculation. Are the images of nurses in high and popular culture different? Have young women been reading popular works, such as the Sue Barton and Cherry Ames series about nursing, that gave them more positive images of nurses than those in the canon? Are there strata in the canon? Are there differences between men's perceptions of nurses and women's perceptions of nurses? What are nursing students and nurses today reading? And what are nursing leaders reading? Finally, does it matter what anyone is reading now that television has become such an omnipresent dispenser of popular images? These are some of the questions provoked by these four essays.

Part II opens with Leslie A. Fiedler's "Images of the Nurse in Fiction and Popular Culture," in which he examines the mythic archetypes of women that still underlie contemporary stereotypes of nurses. He argues that these stereotypes, although modified by the emergence of nursing as a profession a century and a half ago, continue to exert a powerful influence on the deep psyche of the mass audience. Fiedler develops his argument by looking at literary works of Charles Dickens, Walt Whitman, Ernest Hemingway, Robert Heinlein, and Ken Kesey. He pays special attention to the character of Sairey Gamp in Dickens's 1844 novel *Martin Chuzzlewit* because she was the best-known literary image of a nurse until Kesey's 1962 novel *One Flew over the Cuckoo's Nest* gave us Nurse Ratched, whom we still love to hate.

The next essay, Kathryn Montgomery Hunter's "Nurses: The Satiric Image and the Translocated Ideal," is based on the theory that almost all satire reveals or implies an ideal from which the reality it satirizes departs. Thus, the satirical images of women nurses that are so prevalent in literature are countered by literary portraits of good nurses, who are all men. These ideal portraits of (male) nurses Hunter finds in the literary works of five men, Lord Byron, Walt Whitman, Leo Tolstoy, Hart Crane, and Ken Kesey, all of whom write about men nursing other men. Like Fiedler, Hunter focuses much of her attention on Kesey's *One Flew over the Cuckoo's Nest,* but her analysis and conclusion are quite different from his.

Barbara Melosh's essay, "'A Special Relationship': Nurses and Patients in Twentieth-Century Short Stories," begins by examining the relationship between literature and life. After providing this important background, Melosh discusses three recurring themes—power and inequality between nurse and patient, illness as a test of character, and the costs and rewards of caring—as they affect the image of nurse characters in fifteen short stories by such authors as Mary Ellen Chase, F. Scott Fitzgerald, Brendan Gill, Ellen Glasgow, William Goyen, Nancy Hale, William Kotzwinkle, Dorothy Parker, and Frank Tuohy. In Melosh's essay, for the first time in this section, images of nurses created by women authors are held up for scrutiny next to those created by men. In these works by women, the relationships between female nurses and female patients are strikingly different from the relationships between female nurses and male patients, which are the more usual fictional fare.

Part II closes with Joanne Trautmann Banks's "Votaries of Life: Patrick

White's Round-the-Clock Nurses," an analysis of White's 1974 novel *The Eye of the Storm*. Definitely highbrow, this challenging novel presents three nurses who are mythic rather than stereotypic, Banks argues, thus bringing us back to the archetypes Fiedler describes. More important, Banks examines how, in White's novel, nursing's daily chores are transformed into something radiant—a miraculous transcendence of the physical facts of bodily decay to a spiritual realm beyond. Recalling the earlier image of nurse as nun, White's ideal nurse is more secular and existential than religious. His transcendent images of nursing remind us of the important spiritual values of nursing, and of the potential of nursing to lead its best practitioners to the authenticity and transcendent meaning that most people yearn for but rarely attain.

Leslie A. Fiedler

4. Images of the Nurse in Fiction and Popular Culture*

All sub-communities (ethnic, generational, sexual, professional) which constitute the total community of humankind are perceived by others through certain grids of perception perpetuated in literature: myths or stereotypes which more often than not they themselves find offensive— not merely slanderous but objectively "untrue," i.e., unlike certain more favorable images through which they would prefer to be perceived. I was reminded of this the other day when I read in the letter columns of my local newspaper a heartfelt protest from a Registered Nurse which began, "When the ward nurse comes up in conversation, what do you think of? Do images of Mary Benjamin, Hot Lips Houlihan and Nurse Ripples come to mind? Or do you think of the harried young woman with blood spattered on her uniform who answered the call light the last time you or your loved one was hospitalized?"

Quite clearly, the mind of the protestor herself is, like the minds of all the rest of us, possessed by the stereotypes she resents. And how could it be otherwise, since we are all bombarded day and night, so unremittingly that after a while we are scarcely aware of it, by movie and TV versions of the Nurse which are themselves as much "facts" of our experience as actual Nurses themselves. Indeed, there is scarcely anything on the tube these days in which such images do not appear. I am thinking not only of "Doctor Shows" from "Dr. Kildare" and "Marcus Welby, M.D." to "House Calls" and "Nurse," which seem in fact to be losing favor these days, but of continuing series spunoff from earlier films, like "M*A*S*H," which has become everyone's favorite (making Hot Lips perhaps the best known

*Reprinted with permission of Leslie A. Fiedler, State University of New York Press, and The Johns Hopkins University Press, from *Literature and Medicine* 2 (1983):79–90. Copyright © 1983 by State University of New York. Copyright © 1985 by The Johns Hopkins University Press.

Nurse figure of all time), along with the sit-coms and cop shows which possess the small screen after dark, and especially the serial stories, the so-called "Soaps," which preempt the daylight hours on television.

In the latter, nurses are omnipresent; since their typical setting is an enclosed space, and the feelings in which they specialize are pain, suffering and bereavement. What more appropriate then to the form (rivalled only by the bedroom, the courtroom and the prison cell) than the sickroom or the hospital. Indeed, as everyone is aware, the most popular of all daytime serials at the moment is actually called "General Hospital." Moreover, since the audience for such shows is largely—though not, of course, exclu-sively—women, many of their main characters are women, some of them inevitably Nurses; since an archetypal, *the* archetypal female profession has long been nursing—as the names by which its practitioners are called clearly reveal. "Nurse," after all, signifies "nurturer," "milk-giver"; which is to say, Mother or surrogate mother. And the alternative title used by the English, "Sister," complicates the matter even further with associations ecclesiastical or familial, but always female.

In the popular mind, the deep psyche of the mass audience, not merely (in contempt of the changing facts of the case) does Nurse equal Woman, but, on an even profounder mythological level, Woman equals Nurse. But this means that many ancient (male) stereotypes of females in general are transferred automatically to the specific category of nurses. The latter are, in any case, portrayed as being still what some women assuming less tra-ditional female roles refuse to be, subordinate to men: faithful executors of their orders, passive and willingly subordinate. They are, therefore, in their role of sustainers and supporters presented sympathetically, as, say, women business executives, who also appear on the Soaps, are typi-cally not.

But it is not quite as simple as this. After all, nurses preside at the bedsides of males—privileged, even required, unlike other members of their sex, except for prostitutes, to touch, handle, manipulate the naked flesh of males. And they tend, therefore, to be portrayed also as erotic figures of a peculiar, ambiguous kind. They are, that is to say, presented as being at once theoretically taboo (this their uniforms declare, white, cool, starched, reminiscent of the habits of Nuns pledged to eternal chas-tity); and, or at least so the lubricious dreams of the opposite sex have always insisted, not merely sexually desirable, but available, ready and will-ing. Certainly, the line about nurses as potential dates in the movie version of *Marty,* "Money in the bank," evokes the stereotype of their being always at the point of tumbling into the sack, whether to win the heart of a well-heeled patient, or to achieve upward social mobility by marrying a doctor, or simply out of sheer, uninhibited lust. In any case, in the popular arts, nurses are typically portrayed as pursued by or pursuing patients, making passes at or being approached by interns or residents.

But even this is not quite the whole story; since nurses—no longer young and nubile, but grown older, portlier, and more severe as they have been promoted from neophytes to Head Nurses—are no longer imagined as sexually vulnerable sisters but rather equivocal asexual mothers. Sometimes they are conceived as Good Mamas, but more often as Bad ones: bullying, blustering or condescending to the full grown men helpless in their hands ("It's time for us to take our medication. Why don't you sit up tall like a good boy?"), as if they were dependent children. We all of us (women as well as men) lived once as infants and toddlers under a total matriarchy; and men especially have nightmares of regressing to that state of total dependence, nightmares likely to recur in a hospital bed and inevitably projected upon the attendant nurse.

Obviously, all of these stereotypes of the nurse, endlessly reiterated on the screen large or small, existed long before movies or television. Indeed, the archetypes which underlie them are older even than the profession of nursing, as old as patriarchal society itself. But they were profoundly modified by the emergence of that profession some hundred and fifty years ago, when they were fixed in certain "classic" books which we still read, and in more recent ones, which transmit still stereotypes created in the Age of Victoria. Less ephemeral and more respectable than TV shows or Class B movies, such books are preserved in libraries and assigned in classrooms—giving them a special kind of authority. I shall, therefore, from this point on be referring chiefly to them; concentrating, indeed, on those which I have myself at one point or other required of my own students, or have written about in critical studies.

First, however, I feel obliged to mention in passing certain works of non-fiction, which have mythologized the lives and achievement of actual Nurses. Some of these accounts were written as deliberate public relations releases for the still struggling profession, some as propaganda for political causes associated with that profession only because of its mutually beneficial connection with the modern military establishments of various nation states. It was such literature which helped to create favorable images of nurses in the course of turning two major figures, Florence Nightingale and Edith Cavell, first into celebrities and then into legends.

Both were combat nurses, tending wounded troops as only male order-lies had in earlier times—and both were, of course, British. Yet both be-came known worldwide almost immediately. Cavell, to be sure, was a participant in the first war general enough to be called a World War; but Nightingale took part in a limited parochial engagement, the ill-fated English attempt to invade the Crimea. Yet a couple of generations of girls were called "Florence" after Nightingale, and a mountain in Western New York still bears the name of Cavell. It was perhaps the rising tide of femi-nism (though Nightingale was strongly anti-feminist, declaring herself "brutally indifferent" to the plight of women *qua* women), or simply the need for female heroes in a time when only men were actual warriors which explains their appeal.

Certainly it was not the literary quality of the documents which at-tempted to glorify them; since these are by and large shameless schlock produced by nameless hacks, whose appeal was based on values that have since become suspect to anyone with the slightest degree of sophistication. Most of us indeed—several wars later and in a time of revulsion from jingoism of all sorts—are more likely to be embarrassed than moved by the illustrated tracts showing Edith Cavell going down before the bullets of a German firing squad: a martyr to the brutality of the Dirty Huns, the *sales Boches* whom our forefathers and mothers loved to hate. Actually, Cavell was executed after a reasonably fair war crimes trial at the hands of the German Army, accused (on the basis of convincing evidence) of col-laboration with the Belgian Underground and British Intelligence, while using her nurse's role as cover. Her last words, moreover, were reportedly "Patriotism is not enough": a disconcerting remark which was kept an official secret until the time of maximum pacifism between two Great Wars. Small wonder, then, that the literature which created it has disap-peared, though the myth of Cavell as Martyr Nurse somehow survives.

We continue to reprint, however, in more scholarly later biographies, the earliest sentimental-patriotic-heroic accounts of Florence Nightin-gale's mission to the troops of the Crimea, which established in the mind of the world the image of the Nurse as "The Lady with a Lamp," a source of Light in the gathering Darkness. Yet we tend to read them with the same amused condescension as we do the verses she inspired from the Pop poets of her time (admirably sincere but hopelessly inept):

She prays for the dying, she gives peace to the brave,
She feels that the soldier has a soul to be saved,

The wounded they love her as it has been seen.
She's the soldier's preserver, they call her the Queen.
May God give her strength, and her heart never fail,
One of Heaven's best gifts is Miss Nightingale.

It is ironical enough that her image as the nurse *par excellence* has survived nationalism, imperialism and simpleminded missionary zeal, as well as the taste for such poetry. But even more ironical is the fact that similar favorable images of the profession are preserved only in the sub-literature which celebrates those values; these days in novels intended for subteens of all ages, books with titles like *Doctor Gregory's Debutante Nurse, Nurse Ann's Dream Doctor, Theatre Sister in Love, Mink on My Apron* and, of course, *Hold the Lamp High* and *Reluctant Nightingale.* More serious books, however, which is to say, books taken seriously by critics and schoolteachers, are likely still to deal with nurses, as they always have, at worst negatively, at best equivocally.

One of the most wicked of all such wicked caricatures of nurses is the very first—or in any case the earliest still in print and listed under the sub-category of "nurses" in classified bibliographies of fiction. I am referring, of course, to Sairey Gamp, who made her appearance in Charles Dickens's *Martin Chuzzlewit,* initially published in book form in 1844: the very year in which Florence Nightingale finally decided—hearing mysterious voices from heaven—to dedicate herself to a career of nursing. *Martin Chuzzlewit* is not currently one of the favorite novels of Dickens, having been replaced in critical favor by *David Copperfield, Great Expectations,* even *Hard Times.* But I myself have always admired it for its malicious portrayal of mid-nineteenth-century America, its oleaginous villain, Pecksniff, and especially for that large, slovenly, voracious, drunken, endlessly garrulous guardian of the childbed, the sickroom and the mortuary, Mrs. Gamp. Along with an imaginary companion and interlocutor, she is introduced as a minor character, but threatens finally to take over the whole of the book, though she remains peripheral to its main plot.

What she reflects clearly is Dickens's attitude toward nurses, both amateur, which she is in fact, and "professional," which she outrageously claims to be, though she is the very antitype of everything Florence Nightingale dreamed that profession might become. When she is not shamelessly neglecting her patients, she is sadistically punching them, strangling them—presumably in an attempt to induce them to ingest medication; or pushing them closer and closer to the open fire in an effort to "soothe their minds" by a kind of shock treatment that verges on burning them alive. Meanwhile, she is cadging food, drink and hand-me-down clothes and, of course, talking, talking, talking . . .

Scandalous as this portrait may be, it can scarcely be denied that it is in some ways "true to life," i.e., a fair representation of what many, perhaps most, nurses were before the reforms of Nightingale and other Christian Ladies bent on redeeming nursing from its original plebeian practitioners. As a matter of fact, Dickens had actually cleaned up Sairey a little, presumably to avoid shocking his genteel audience; portraying her, that is to say, as a celibate though alcoholic widow rather than a prostitute and/or bawd, as indeed many such early Victorian nurses were.

What intrigues us still about Sairey Gamp, however, is the mythic nightmare figure which persists just beneath her "realistic," satiric surfaces, and the archaic fears of Woman as Witch which that figure embodies. Typically unconscious in writer and reader alike, those fears provide a clue to the hostility toward nurses which popular literature strives to conceal by sentimentalizing and idealization, and books like Dickens's try to exorcise with ridicule. It pays to notice in this light just what it is that Mrs. Gamp *does*. Not only does she provide bedside care for the sick, day and night; but she also delivers babies and prepares corpses for burial. Lying-in and laying-out are still her province, as they were the province of women exclusively before the patriarchal revolution which turned them over to "professional" male obstetricians and funeral directors. Only the tending of the ill (perhaps because it is the least terrifying and taboo of the original threefold functions) was left to women.

Sairey Gamp, however, still practises all three of the traditional mysteries of life and death originally associated, along with the expurgated final mystery of Sex, with the Great Mother, the White Goddess; and which, after the emergence of patriarchal deities, survived in the underground religion as the province of the "Wise Women" or Witches. It is in any case as a Witch, albeit a comic one, that Sairey Gamp is portrayed: one in whose unclean hands all three traditional functions turn malign. Not only does her actual practise travesty the role of bedside healer to which she lays claim; but even more as midwife and layer-out of the dead her skills are shown as debouching in mutilation and monstrosity. Early on in the novel, we hear her talking of her first corpse, her own husband, whom she describes as stretched out stark and cold "with a penny-piece on each eye, and his wooden leg under his left arm. . . ."[1] And toward the end, she recounts having come on her imaginary friend's "sweet infant . . . kep in spirits in a bottle . . . " and therefore displayed in a travelling show of freaks "in company with the pink-eyed lady, Prooshan dwarf, and livin' skelinton . . . " (p. 893).

But Dickens wants to have it both ways: evoking contempt from his readers for the persistence in Mrs. Gamp as Nurse of what is still archaic (still resistant to the rationalization and hierarchization of the medical profession), but also for her claims to absolute authority in the sickroom in the name of professionalism. In chapter headings and in the text, Dickens uses the word "professional" over and over as a term of contempt; making it clear that he objects not only to the shamanistic past of Nursing but to the scientific, bureaucratic future imagined for it by Florence Nightingale. Not that he is opposed to demystification; but what he advocates is humanization rather than professionalization or certification. This he makes clear in the parting words of advice given by Old Martin Chuzzlewit to a discomfited Mrs. Gamp, ". . . a little less liquor, and a little more humanity, and a little less regard for herself, and a little more regard for her patients, and perhaps a trifle of additional honesty" (p. 894).

In any case, Dickens's two-pronged indictment of nurses suggests a double bind, a no-win situation for the profession, out of which—at least in the imagination of the makers of our most respected books—they still struggle in vain to extricate themselves. Certainly, this is true of Ken Kesey's *One Flew over the Cuckoo's Nest*, published more than a century after *Martin Chuzzlewit*, in 1962. In that novel, Kesey created the character of Nurse Ratched, the most memorable mythological portrait of a nurse since Sairey Gamp; and it is therefore with a discussion of it that I propose to conclude. But there are certain works which appeared in the years between which demand to be mentioned in passing, though none of them possesses equal archetypal resonance.

The first is an extraordinary poem by the greatest of American poets, the only major writer to deal with nurses who had actually been a nurse— a combat nurse, in fact, quite like Florence Nightingale and Edith Cavell. This was, of course, Walt Whitman, who just after the end of the American Civil War (once more in the reign of Queen Victoria) added to his continually revised epic, *Leaves of Grass,* a section called "Drum-Taps," at the very center of which stands "The Wound-Dresser." From the beginning of his career as a poet, Whitman had been possessed by an image of himself as a comforter of the afflicted, a healing presence at the bedside of the sick; writing, for instance, in "The Sleepers," one of the twelve poems published in the first edition of *Leaves of Grass,* "I stand in the dark with drooping eyes by the worst-suffering and the most restless, / I pass my hands soothingly to and fro a few inches from them, / The restless sink in their beds, they fitfully sleep."[2]

During the Civil War, however, Whitman actually tended the wounded in military hospitals in Washington, D.C., turning fantasy into fact and fact back into poetry:

Bearing the bandages, water and sponge,
Straight and swift to my wounded I go,
Where they lie on the ground after the battle brought in,
Where their priceless blood reddens the grass the ground,
....

From the stump of the arm, the amputated hand,
I undo the clotted lint, remove the slough, wash off the matter and
    blood,
Back on his pillow the soldier bends with curv'd neck and side-
    falling head,
His eyes are closed, his face is pale, he dares not look on the bloody
    stump,
And has not yet look'd on it.
....

I dress the perforated shoulder, the foot with the bullet-wound,
Cleanse the one with a gnawing and putrid gangrene, so sickening,
    so offensive,
While the attendant stands behind aside me holding the tray and
    pail.

I am faithful, I do not give out,
The fractur'd thigh, the knee, the wound in the abdomen,
These and more I dress with impassive hand, (yet deep in my
    breast a fire, a burning flame.)

Thus in silence in dreams' projections,
Returning, resuming, I thread my way through the hospitals,
The hurt and wounded I pacify with soothing hand,
I sit by the restless all the dark night, some are so young,
Some suffer so much, I recall the experience sweet and sad,

(Many a soldier's loving arms about this neck have cross'd and
   rested,
Many a soldier's kiss dwells on these bearded lips.)[3]

Most people, however, remembering images of nurses in literature do
not recall this poem, in part because Whitman was of the wrong gender,
a male pretender to a role which mythologically we associate with the
female of the species. Moreover, his vision of the *eros* of nursing, the sexual
overtones of the bedside encounter with the maimed and the wounded, is
disturbingly ambiguous, containing hints of lubricity and sado-maso-
chism compatible neither with the benign popular cliché of the nurse as a
sexless secular saint, nor the Gamp anti-stereotype of an equally sexless
though malevolent exploiter of her patients. Equally disconcerting to the
readers of Whitman's own time—and to many still, even in our "enlight-
ened" age—are the homosexual implications of his verses. Nonetheless,
"The Wound-Dresser" remains the most moving and subtle evocation in
print of the experience of nursing in a time of war—*from the viewpoint of
the nurse*.

When, however, some fifty years later, in Ernest Hemingway's *A Farewell to Arms,* another American writer, out of his own experience in another major war, attempted to evoke (this time in prose) the figure of the
nurse, it was from the viewpoint of the *nursed.* Unlike Whitman, Hemingway, though he was not a combatant (serving as a volunteer with the Italian Ambulance Corps) was also not a nurse. Moreover, he reimagines his
semi-autobiographical protagonist, Lieutenant Henry, as a soldier who
after being drastically wounded, manages to survive World War I to tell
his tale. It is his nurse, Catherine Barkley, who dies—as seems at first im-
probable but finally appropriate enough in a time haunted by the legend
of Edith Cavell, who was killed in the midst of combat. Catherine, however, does not like the latter die at the hands of a German firing squad but
in childbirth; condemned by her author, for reasons best known to himself, to meet her end in the hospital where she has gone hoping to produce
new life.

Finally, the figure of Catherine Barkley, however pathetic, remains too
conventional, too like the Pop stereotype of the nurse to remain in our
conscious minds, much less to haunt our dreams. Passive, obedient, utterly
subject to the wills of her medical superiors and her lover, wanting desperately to be "a good girl" but unable to deny the wounded soldier her
bed, she provides an erotic alternative to the thanatic desolation of war.

But somehow we never quite believe in her. Indeed, there is a kind of critical consensus that there is only one real rounded character in Hemingway's novel, Henry himself; the rest, including Catherine, are ghosts even before they die.

Moreover, just as in *A Farewell to Arms* Catherine produced no viable offspring, so also as literary prototype she inspired no notable protagonists in the best loved fiction of the thirties, forties, and fifties, either best sellers or art novels. Not, in fact, until the late sixties, the period of the Counter Culture, did the nurse re-emerge as a central figure; this time in the cult literature of the young—particularly in two underground favorites, Robert Heinlein's *Stranger in a Strange Land* and Ken Kesey's *One Flew over the Cuckoo's Nest*.

It is, however, almost impossible to remember that the major female character in *Stranger in a Strange Land* is a nurse, despite the fact that Heinlein announces in the opening pages that "Gillian Boardman was a competent nurse and her hobby was men."[4] Moreover, when the male protagonist, who has been brought up on Mars, arrives on Earth weak and helpless as a baby, she bustles about his hospital bed, speaking in the regal first person plural as we have learned from TV shows all nurses do, "Well, how are we today? Feeling better?" (p. 20). Before the book's end, however, even the author seems to have forgotten her profession, letting her blend into the scarcely individualized gaggle of good lays, the secretaries, sideshow entertainers and strippers, who constitute the whole of his female cast. Indeed, eventually Gillian becomes a stripper, too, and at last an avatar of the Earth Goddess, the incarnation of female sexuality in the half-fraudulent ritual of a communal cult, in which all the men possess all the women turn and turn about. She represents, that is to say, little more than the ancient cliché of the nurse as erotic object raised to its highest power; and she tends to fade therefore from the memories of those who read the book in quest of something up-to-date: an advocacy of cannibalism, let's say, or of sex without commitment or guilt.

Heinlein's was the first work of avowed science fiction to become a best-seller, and it continues to be reprinted more than twenty years later. But though it has added a new verb to the language ("to grok") and provided rituals for Charles Manson's murderous "religion," none of its women characters are of truly mythic dimensions—certainly not its single nurse. Such an authentically archetypal character did appear, however, in an even more brutally misogynous novel published at about the same time, *One Flew over the Cuckoo's Nest,* which takes place in the psychiatric ward of the State Hospital, presided over by a monster in female form known as Nurse Ratched, or more familiarly, "Big Nurse." That larger-than-life tyrant of the ward does not quite attain the full archetypal dimensions of other memorable women in our literature, Hester Prynne, for instance (who, I remind you, ends up playing a nursely role in the community that casts her out) or even Scarlett O'Hara (who fails miserably in her attempt to become a Civil War wound-dresser *à la* Walt Whitman). Yet she has become a byword and a myth over the twenty years since her first appearance—replacing Sairey Gamp for the contemporary reader as the mythic nurse *par excellence*.

But how different she is from her predecessor: not slovenly but neat to a fault—encased in ironed and starched white garb, spotless, unspottable. Moreover, far from being a drunk, she is the enemy of booze, even as she is the enemy of sexual promiscuity, gambling, all hedonism and moral looseness. A super-professional rather than a helpless amateur, she is organized and the organizer of everyone around her: just such an efficient administrator, in fact, as Florence Nightingale dreamed and became. Though she is not portrayed as a combat nurse, we are told that Ratched has learned her trade, grown old and rigid while serving in the army—finally introjecting the values of the modern military into the routine of the hospital, as Nightingale also dreamed that nurses of the future might do.

But Big Nurse remains for Kesey hateful still, even more hateful in fact; since she is no longer comic and cannot be laughed away, anymore than she can be brought into line (as Mrs. Gamp could still be) by a threat to call the police. She has become the police; and can therefore only be subdued through an act of outlawry, like the rapist's murderous assault, vain but gallant, made on her by the book's major male character, R. P. McMurphy. In part Kesey's attitude can be explained by the age which bred him and whose spokesman he became: a revolutionary time, when all hierarchal institutions, not least the hospital, had come to be despised, and all professions, specialties—especially, perhaps, medical ones, and most especially psychiatry—were regarded with hostility and suspicion. After all, in the late sixties, as reading R. D. Laing reminds us, madness had come to be venerated in many quarters as a higher kind of sanity.

But disconcertingly, Big Nurse is also hated and feared for what she has in common with Mrs. Gamp: i.e., because she is a woman; and the equation of woman and nurse persists in the deep male psyche still despite superficial changes in the profession. For McMurphy, her attempt to "cure" psychosis, i.e., force all psychological deviants into conformity with the system, seems a kind of ball-breaking: a war against manhood, which beginning with the administration of tranquillizers, moves on to electroshock therapy and reveals its true motive which it climaxes in lobotomy—that ultimate form of castration. To Kesey, indeed, all women—except possibly prostitutes—represent Bad Mama, which is to say, mother after she has withdrawn the breast (and Nurse Ratched is portrayed as the biggest titted white mother of them all under her starched uniform) and taken up the rod. Freedom, therefore, is to be found only in a constant flight from them and all they represent. Otherwise the American male is doomed to end up a cog in the machine, like most of the great world outside the asylum, a self-castrated victim like Billy Bibbit, or a mere vegetable like McMurphy after his failed attempt to reach the living flesh beneath Ratched's pristine whites.

Such attitudes are based on a special American brand of *machismo* and misogyny much older than the Cultural Revolution, as old, indeed, as our literature itself, beginning with the revolt of Rip Van Winkle against what Washington Irving called "petticoat tyranny." In this view, women—especially White women, imbued with the values of European Christianity—represent not what Sairey Gamp still symbolized for Dickens: the anarchy of the unconscious, the primordial and the archaic, but consciousness, conscience, repression: what Huck Finn, about to flee into the Wilderness, calls "civilization." It seems inevitable in light of this that when nurses have ceased to be thought of as vestigial witches and are re-imagined as machine tenders, soulless machines themselves, it be an American author who bestows on them their new mythological name.

What is baffling is that the American public, male and female, continues to hate Nurse Ratched and to love McMurphy for his failed assault on her, not merely as they live on in the still reprinted novel but as they have been reborn in the late seventies in an immensely successful movie. What our response betrays is the persistence of attitudes we like to think of ourselves as having long outgrown not just toward nurses but toward all women whom that profession still mythologically represents. And perhaps, after all, it is the function of literature to remind us (though for better or for worse who can say?) of precisely such otherwise unconfessed impulses; the dark side of our ambivalence toward both those who bear us and those who tend us when we are ill.

Notes

1. Charles Dickens, *The Life and Adventures of Martin Chuzzlewit* (Harmonds-worth, England: Penguin Books, 1968), 378. All subsequent page references are to this edition and will be cited parenthetically in the text.
2. Walt Whitman, "The Sleepers," lines 23–25, from *Leaves of Grass* (1855), in Walt Whitman, *Complete Poetry and Collected Prose,* ed. Justin Kaplan (New York: Library of America, 1982), 543.
3. Walt Whitman, "The Wound-Dresser," lines 25–28, 45–49, 53–65, from *Leaves of Grass* (1891–92), in Walt Whitman, *Complete Poetry and Collected Prose,* ed. Justin Kaplan (New York: Library of America, 1982), 443–45.
4. Robert A. Heinlein, *Stranger in a Strange Land* (New York: Berkley, 1968), 19. All subsequent page references are to this edition and will be cited parenthetically in the text.

Kathryn Montgomery Hunter

5. Nurses: The Satiric Image and the Translocated Ideal*

The contemporary crisis of identity experienced by the nursing profession is to some extent a part of the larger predicament shared by all women. What is the social value of care?—child care, care of the elderly, care of the ill and dying? Who is to do it and how are they to be esteemed and rewarded?

At first glance literature might seem to have little to offer to an analysis of this problem. Literary images are not isomorphic with social reality,[1] and nowhere is this more true than with the literary image of the nurse. She is sentimentalized, romanticized, satirized, but seldom presented straightforwardly. A character who is a nurse in fiction or drama is immediately symbolic. Her profession has been given her for a thematic purpose. She could not become, in midstory (as friends in midlife have), a lawyer or a minister or a health-care policy expert. A nurse is who she is. She is a metaphor for all women and for the problems posed for men by women. If women's problematic submissiveness is at issue, who better focuses this than a nurse? If assertiveness is the complication, nurses are among those who, when assertive, are most threatening. Although common sense or a few days in a hospital might suggest other fictional possibilities, in literature a nurse is never not symbolic.

This gap between fictional image and social reality is readily apparent, of course, in the popular culture that Leslie Fiedler so well describes.[2] But it exists, too, in "high" literature. In the works of the past two centuries most likely to appear on a high school or college reading list,[3] works written for the most part by men, the strongest portraits of nurses are caricatures: drunken, disheveled Sairey Gamp in Charles Dickens's *Martin Chuzzlewit* (1844), castrating Nurse Ratched in Ken Kesey's *One Flew over*

*With thanks to Joseph Cady, New York City.

the Cuckoo's Nest (1962), man-hating Jenny Field in John Irving's *The World According to Garp* (1978).[4] The same body of literature offers only a few attractive portraits of those who care for the ill. These gentle, noninvasive, caring nurses are, quite surprisingly, men.

Such an unexpected polarity between good nurses who are men and the prevailing satiric image of nurses who are women no doubt suggests something about the state of antifeminism in our culture and how it manifests itself. Nursing was not an organized profession until late in the nineteenth century; it was scarcely even a specialized group. Instead, the care of the ill and the newborn and the dead was the duty of us all—or that half of us who are women. The sexes participate in the mind-body duality—may even be the ideational source of it. Women are associated intimately with the body, and therefore, with weakness and fallibility and temptation. We are responsible for birth and sex and health and cleanliness—and illness and death. For men the loss of control, the regression into helplessness experienced by the ill,[5] is also a loss of what might be called manhood. Pain, fear, loneliness, all the things that we all hope to avoid in life, are for them an additional loss of power in the world. Their submission to a regimen and to a (usually female) person who enforces it is required before they can return to the world. This has its pleasant side, of course: attention, care, encouragement, recovery. But it is also a reminder, a harbinger of mortality and of the subservience of the body to time and death. Women also may feel restive and rebellious under a nurse's care; there is Katherine Anne Porter's heroine in "Pale Horse, Pale Rider," for example. But her frustration is not with her powerlessness, but, on the contrary, with being dragged back into life.

Is illness different for women patients? I believe it is. We had people of our own sex as our caretakers in childhood; men had nurturers of the opposite sex.[6] While their coming into adulthood and independence may for that reason be more complete and apparently achieved, it is nevertheless more abrupt and radical. They will not be mothers; they are exiled from all that. Our culture is not so radically antifeminist as the fifth- and fourth-century Athenian one described by Philip Slater,[7] but we come close. There, boys were sequestered with their mothers and sisters till the age of seven, when they were "rescued" by their fathers and taken out into the city to learn their lives as citizens. Slater links this to the hostility of Greek goddesses toward mortal males. As southern whites so amply demonstrated,[8] human beings fear and hate and attribute fantastic powers to those whom they repress and control. A similar attitude toward women finds its lightning rod in chastely uniformed nurses whose profession is intimate service.

Nurse Ratched, the Big Nurse who rules over the mental ward in Ken Kesey's *One Flew over the Cuckoo's Nest,* is often said to represent the contemporary image of nursing, despite the novel's origin in the gynophobic 1950s. A close look reveals that she is much more: she is a representative of women and the roles assigned us. She is first of all a mother—and not only "a mother"[9] with the borrowed black street pronunciation that the hero McMurphy gives the word. To Chief Bromden, the novel's narrator, she represents society, the "'Combine,' which is a huge organization that aims to adjust the Outside as well as she has the Inside. . . ."[10] "Practice," he says, "has steadied and strengthened her until now she wields a sure power that extends in all directions on hairlike wires too small for anybody's eye but mine; I see her sit in the center of this web of wires like a watchful robot, tend her network with mechanical insect skill, know every second which wire runs where and just what current to send up to get the results she wants" (p. 30). This is paranoia, of course, but we are meant to understand that disorder in Chief Bromden is a matter of metaphor taken literally, as reality.[11] His vision of Big Nurse is Kesey's and is meant to be ours.

Women are not merely accidentally or partially or even indirectly the villains in *One Flew over the Cuckoo's Nest,* as a comparison with the black characters in the book will show. Kesey's auxiliary villains are the three "black boys," with "eyes glittering out of the black faces like the hard glitter of radio tubes out of the back of an old radio" (p. 9). Specialists in sadism and sodomy, they and the mousey, compliant psychiatrist make up the Big Nurse's "ideal staff." Nevertheless, it would be difficult to call Kesey a racist precisely because these three owe their evil to the system that co-opts them:

> The first one she gets five years after I been on the ward [Chief Bromden tells us], a twisted sinewy dwarf the color of cold asphalt. His mother was raped in Georgia while his papa stood by tied to the hot iron stove with plow traces, blood streaming into his shoes. The boy watched from a closet, five years old . . . and he never grew an inch after. . . . He wanted to carry a sock full of birdshot when he first came on the job, to work the patients into shape, but she told him they didn't do it that way anymore, made him leave the sap at home and taught him her own technique. . . . (pp. 31–32)

The other two are tall and thin: "their faces are chipped into expressions that never change, like flint arrowheads. Their eyes come to points. If you brush against their hair it rasps the hide right off you" (p. 32). The Big Nurse hones their anger to suit her orderly repressive needs. They are villains, agents of evil, but the sources of their evil are damning to society and its racism. They stand justified in the world of the novel. They are, like those they victimize, victims of the Combine.

There is, in addition, one sympathetic black keeper, just as there is one briefly glimpsed sympathetic nurse. He is old and addressed as Mister; she is young and Japanese and offers the only explanation for Nurse Ratched's character and behavior: she is an old army nurse, used to having her own way. In the absence of any explanation in cultural or political terms for women's behavior and social roles, including Nurse Ratched's, this is no explanation at all. Women in this novel are not the creatures of society; society is theirs,[12] and the Big Nurse is their epitome.

She is a large-breasted but asexual woman with a face like "white enamel" (p. 129) and a voice like a saw (p. 127). Our first knowledge of her is curiously sexual: hers is the key, "soft and swift and familiar," that locks cleave to (p. 10). She is an "angel of mercy" in the patient Harding's ironic description (p. 57), just like a mother, who, as she is fond of telling "her" ward, acts and punishes "*entirely* for your own good" (p. 171). She exercises power over doctors; aspiring residents fear her; her ward runs like well-oiled machinery. All men return to childhood in her presence, all but Randle P. McMurphy. Other women in the novel are equally stereotypical if not quite so symbolic. Harding's homosexuality is shameful to him principally because of the torment his wife puts him to; another character mutters only "fuck da wife"; Billy Bibbit's mother, a seductive smotherer straight out of Philip Wylie's *Generation of Vipers* (1942), has had him locked up in an insane asylum rather than acknowledge his adulthood, which is to say, his sexuality. Chief Bromden's mother, a white woman whose last name he bears, belittled his father, The-Pine-That-Stands-Tallest-on-the-Mountain, until he became too "little" to defend the rights of his tribe (p. 187). Women that are depicted as attractive are the fifteen-year-old "little hooker" that caught McMurphy on a charge of statutory rape, the women on his pack of playing cards, and the fresh, honest heart-of-gold girls from Portland—"Who cares how they make their living?"—who understand and enjoy their place in this scheme. The other nurses are called "the little nurses," perhaps descriptively, perhaps condescendingly, probably both. The most painful of these creatures is the night nurse, wrung with anxiety, a birthmark on her face and crucifix helpless between her breasts.

Men are different. Even in an insane asylum. McMurphy, when he arrives, smells fascinatingly of sweat and work (p. 91). "Man" can represent the whole human race in the first half of the narrator's sentence, then be used again in the second half in its sexual sense. Of the Chronics on the morning of the big fishing trip with the legendary "two whores from Portland," Chief Bromden says: "They could know because enough of the man in them had been damped out that the old animal instincts had taken over . . . , and they could be jealous because there was enough man left to still remember" (p. 192). Above all, men laugh. Laughter, once they get the hang of it, makes them powerful, swells them up to full size (p. 212). It is fitting that the final patient rebellion takes place in a comradely common shower, almost a locker room, with Chief Bromden and McMurphy acting as one to defend their buddy from a symbolic rape.

In Kesey's novel—and for the readers who have read it as a manifesto against repressive modern society—nursing is the symbol of female power. It is not a new and forthright, liberating political power, but the old manipulative power of the oppressed, turning the tables, lurking in the intimate corners of life to unman the manly, reducing them to children, to helpless bodies. Women are allied with the uncontrollable that controls us; women are to blame.

But what if nursing were detached from womanhood? There are, as I have suggested, good nurses in literature, gentle, calm tenders of the ill or dying, but with very few exceptions these caretakers are men. Theirs is gratuitous care, freely given, an expression of patriotism or brotherhood or the love of man for men. Their care transcends class boundaries and restores to the ill the dignity that their self-sacrifice in war or their participation in the common fate of all mankind has bestowed on them.

"That must be very unpleasant for you," says Leo Tolstoy's hero in *The Death of Ivan Ilych* (1886) to Gerasim, the butler's young healthy assistant who has taken on the task of carrying out his bedpan.[13] Ivan Ilych is tormented by this necessity, "from the uncleanliness, the unseemliness, and the smell, and from knowing that another person had to take part in it" (p. 135):

> "You must forgive me. I am helpless."
> "Oh, why, sir," [Gerasim replies] . . . , "what's a little trouble? It's a case of illness with you, sir." (p. 136)

Ivan Ilych is comfortable only when his feet are raised. His wife describes the position as one that is no doubt bad for him—such an uncooperative patient, and the doctor smiles "with a contemptuous affability that said: 'What's to be done? These sick people do have foolish fancies of that kind, but we must forgive them'" (p. 142). Only Gerasim does not lie to Ivan Ilych; only Gerasim sees his loneliness and pities him. Ivan Ilych is comfortable only with Gerasim, comforted only by his presence. When he sends the young man away to rest, Gerasim refuses to go: "Don't you worry, Ivan Ilych. I'll get sleep enough later on" (p. 138), acknowledging openly, as no one else will, that it soon will be over. "We shall all of us die, so why should I grudge a little trouble?" (p. 138). Tolstoy comments: ". . . he was doing it for a dying man and hoped someone would do the same for him when his time came" (p. 138).

The same unflinching acceptance of bodily fact is found in Walt Whitman's *Drum-Taps* (1865), a part of *Leaves of Grass* written out of the poet's experience as a nurse with the Union Army. He claims that he had intended to be a soldier, but that at the age of forty-three "resign'd [him]self, / To sit by the wounded and soothe them, or silently watch the dead."[14] The celebration of the body that characterizes his earlier poetry here turns to a cherishing of the injured, often mutilated body and to meditation on the beauty and nobility of the dead. "The Wound-Dresser" is the best known of these poems. Imagining himself asked in old age about his memories of the Civil War, he describes his passage through a field hospital:

> Bearing the bandages, water and sponge,
> Straight and swift to my wounded I go,
>
> . . . .
>
> I am firm with each, the pangs are sharp yet unavoidable,
> One turns to me his appealing eyes—poor boy! I never knew you,
> Yet I think I could not refuse this moment to die for you,
>   if that would save you.   (ll. 25–26, 36–38)

He invokes "sweet death" to take the cavalry-man dying slowly with a bullet through his neck; he dresses the stump of an arm that its owner will not look at:

I dress the perforated shoulder, the foot with the bullet-wound,
Cleanse the one with a gnawing and putrid gangrene, so sickening,
    so offensive,
While the attendant stands behind aside me holding the tray and
    pail.

I am faithful, I do not give out,
The fractur'd thigh, the knee, the wound in the abdomen,
These and more I dress with impassive hand, (yet deep in my
    breast a fire, a burning flame.)   (ll. 53–58)

Whitman's homosexuality is not irrelevant here, but it will not go the whole way toward understanding the poem. The speaker has been a witness to suffering. The wounds he dresses have a historic importance in the life of a nation: the young, he imagines, will ask him in his old age about the experience. Nevertheless, the poem documents again and again the importance of the wounds for the individuals who suffer them. The soldier with the amputated hand is unnamed; we do not know what he looks like. We are told little more about him than the nature of his wound, rather like the situation common in a modern hospital. But that little tells all:

Back on his pillow the soldier bends with curv'd neck and side-
    falling head,
His eyes are closed, his face is pale, he dares not look on the bloody
    stump,
And has not yet look'd on it.   (ll. 47–49)

Whitman's attention to the essential is most apparent when apparently most useless: in the care for the dead. "Vigil Strange I Kept on the Field One Night" is a brief elegy for a young soldier whom the poet returns to find lying dead:

Long there and then in vigil I stood, dimly around me the battle-
    field spreading,
Vigil wondrous and vigil sweet there in the fragrant silent night,
But not a tear fell, not even a long-drawn sigh, long, long I gazed,
Then on the earth partially reclining sat by your side leaning my
    chin in my hands,

Passing sweet hours, immortal and mystic hours with you dearest
   comrade—not a tear, not a word,
Vigil of silence, love and death, vigil for you my son and my
   soldier,
As onward silently stars aloft, eastward new ones upward stole,
Vigil final for you brave boy, (I could not save you, swift was your
   death,
I faithfully loved you and cared for you living, I think we shall
   surely meet again,)[15]

Then, as dawn comes, he wraps the body carefully and buries him "where he fell" (l. 26).

Nurses will notice immediately that there is not much work in this poem; cost-containment programs would short-circuit if this act of care were restored to nursing. But what Whitman the nurse has done is a human necessity, especially in the absence of a family, and he has done it unintrusively, grieving and paying homage to the soldier without retelling his life story or grasping for its meaning. The young man simply was, and now he is no longer. This is difficult and, I believe, unusual. Jorge Luis Borges has described how we survivors customarily rob the dead of the details of their lives, stripping them to abstractions till they are "the loss and absence of the world."[16] Whitman the nurse seems, like Gerasim, to be able to contemplate the dead and dying in all their eponymous individuality even as they participate in common mortality.

In contrast with Whitman, Byron has only one poem of this kind, the posthumously titled and published "Love and Death" (1824). It is a love poem to Loukas Chalandritsanos, his page during the Greek war against the Turks, and each of its stanzas recounts acts of self-sacrifice he has undertaken for the young man's sake. The first three quatrains begin "I watch'd thee . . . ," naming as dangers the war, their shipwreck, and Loukas's illness:

I watch'd thee when the fever glazed thine eyes,
   Yielding my couch and stretch'd me on the ground,
When overworn with watching, ne'er to rise
   From thence if thou an early grave hadst found.[17]

Byron makes no more of it than of his seeking out the young man during an earthquake, but it is this simplicity and naturalness that is remarkable.

Such care is what is due a person one loves, a proof of that love—even when, as in this case, the love is not returned.

A century later Hart Crane's nursing poem, "Episode of Hands" (1948), is politically romantic. It recounts the act of care that is a bond between an injured worker and the factory owner's son:

And as the fingers of the factory owner's son,
That knew a grip for books and tennis
As well as one for iron and leather,—
As his taut, spare fingers wound the gauze
Around the thick bed of the wound,
His own hands seemed to him
Like wings of butterflies
Flickering in sunlight over summer fields.[18]

He admires the scarred toughness of the worker's hand in his:

And factory sounds and factory thoughts
Were banished from him by that larger, quieter hand
That lay in his with the sun upon it.
And as the bandage knot was tightened
The two men smiled into each other's eyes.   (ll. 20–24)

There are more romantic bonds here than the political one, of course. The excuse of physical care shelters the opportunity for socially acceptable physical contact between people of the same sex. This poem raises more clearly than the others the question of how we are to read these works. It will not do to sum them up as homosexual. Tolstoy's is not; the love poem among them was written by a man who had more women lovers than men and is customarily regarded as heterosexual. All participate in a political vision—whether Christian or socialist or nationalist—of liberty, brother-hood, and community. Both Tolstoy and Crane romanticize the lower class, either as a source of health and sane good sense or as a repository of an oppositeness that may redeem even the industrialist. Whitman, who celebrates his love for men most explicitly, has written the poem most explicit about the work of caring for the ill. These are not, then, literary works about nursing that simply disguise a longing to touch safely a body of the same sex. I believe that a longing to give and receive care is primary, and that it is to be found, frustrated, even in *One Flew over the Cuckoo's Nest*. For there, too, the true caretakers are men.

Kesey carefully separates the role of caretaker, the true nurturer, from homosexuality, but he does not separate it from sexuality itself. Although the black boys threaten their charges with sodomy, there is only a modicum of homophobia in the novel. The black boys represent rape. Harding's homosexuality, on the other hand, has made him a victim of society. It has not crippled him, he realizes near the end of the novel; he has rather been made mentally ill by society's condemnation of him. Of his "insanity" he says, "It's society's way of dealing with someone different" (p. 257). McMurphy has helped him to this self-acceptance. Midway in the novel the Chief reports:

> I'd see him [McMurphy] do things that didn't fit with his face or hands, things like painting a picture at OT with real paints on a blank paper with no lines or numbers anywhere on it to tell him where to paint, or like writing letters to somebody in a beautiful flowing hand. . . . Harding had hands that looked like they should have done paintings though they never did; Harding trapped his hands and forced them to work sawing planks for doghouses. McMurphy wasn't like that. He hadn't let what he looked like run his life one way or the other, any more than he'd let the Combine mill him into fitting where they wanted him to fit. (p. 140)

When Billy Bibbit, the thirty-one-year-old virgin, is preparing for his night with Candy, McMurphy teaches him to dance, taking the woman's part, cheerfully enduring the teasing that follows, so that Billy can learn to lead.

The homosexual possibilities in McMurphy's promise to make the Chief "big again" must be heard as plainly as its strategy of appealing to the Chief's habit of literalizing metaphor. His father's loss of stature and power we have understood in both a political and a personal, sexual sense. Yet the possibility is almost defused when McMurphy actually gives the Chief an erection by describing in vivid detail the women who will swoon in his path once he is back to his old, sane, powerful size. McMurphy claims the double entendre for his own:

> And all of a sudden his hand shot out and with a swing of his arm untied my sheet, cleared my bed covers, and left me lying there naked.
> "Look there, Chief. Haw. What'd I tell you? You growed a half a foot already."
> Laughing, he walked down the row of beds to the hall. (p. 190)

The Chief loves him, of course. Earlier in the same scene, the Chief is moved to say his first words in years. McMurphy has laughed at his habit of hiding old rechewed gum underneath his bed, then provoked him miraculously to laughter by singing a chorus of "Does the Spearmint lose its flavor on the bedpost over niiiite?" He concludes by tossing the Chief a package of Juicy Fruit: "And before I realized what I was doing [the Chief says], I told him Thank you" (p. 185). Then with McMurphy waiting for him to talk, "the only thing that came to [his] mind was the kind of thing one man can't say to another because it sounds wrong in words" (p. 185). So it goes unsaid—but not forgotten. When he has told his story in a flood of words and McMurphy lies silent, the Chief thinks perhaps he ought to touch him "to see if he's still alive. . . . ":

> That's a lie. I know he's still alive. That ain't the reason I want to touch him.
> I want to touch him because he's a man.
> That's a lie too. There's other men around. I could touch them.
> I want to touch him because I'm one of these queers!
> But that's a lie too. That's one fear hiding behind another. If I was one of these queers I'd want to do other things with him. I just want to touch him because he's who he is. (p. 188)

The principal caretaker in the novel is McMurphy, who reclaims the Chief and Harding and for a time even Billy Bibbit from the clutches of the Combine. They too learn to care for others. Harding gives up his ironic resignation, accepts his beautiful hands, and urges care and escape on McMurphy. Billy Bibbit learns to dare to give his jacket to Candy and to know he should defend her. The Chief, who recovers his voice and stature and sanity along with the capacity to love, presides over the disposition of McMurphy's body, that "crummy sideshow fake" left after dozens of shock treatments and the final lobotomy. Listening to him breathe again, this time hoping it will stop, the Chief takes up a pillow and "finally had to lie full length on top of it and scissor the kicking legs with [his] while [he] mashed the pillow into the face. [He] lay there on top of the body for what seemed days. Until the thrashing stopped. Until it was still a while and had shuddered once and was still again. Then [he] rolled off" (p. 270). This is an act of love, a parody of a caricature of nursing, as well as the ironic end of social suffocation and oppressive care.

That the true caretakers in *One Flew over the Cuckoo's Nest* are men places the novel in what amounts to a quasi-tradition of works that embody a

translocated ideal of nursing. Almost all satire (Swift is the notable exception) reveals or implies an ideal of human behavior or political organization from which the reality it satirizes departs.[19] It is not that satirists feel
any moral obligation to present a description of the way life ought to be;
it is simply that somewhere in the work there will be a character or an
event that becomes the standard by which we judge the satirized characters
or events or objects. This ideal is violated at least symbolically and perhaps
destroyed in fact by the forces that govern the satiric world.

The ideal violated in satires of nurses is the expectation of undemand-
ing maternal love and care, a demand that quickly extends itself to sexual
compliance. The nurse ought to be the perfect mother, but she fails as
surely as her predecessor did, enforcing rules, saying no. The satiric image
of the nurse focuses anger at mothers, at their failure to be always available
with unconditional attention and love, and, perhaps especially for men, at
their attempts to protect us and forestall our independence and activity in
the world. This anger does not fall exclusively on nurses. It can be gener-
alized to all women, as it is in Kesey's novel, and, for much of human
history before the organization of the nursing profession, it was the lot of
the stepmother. All may be imagined as anti-mothers: manipulative, controlling, noncaring, dangerous, unresponsive, frigid, whores.

In the satire of nurses, in literature generally, where are we likely to find
the ideal of a generous mother-love expressed? The question is almost
absurd. Certainly it won't be in the fictional character's recollections of
infancy: those memories have been superseded by the nay-saying images
that fuel the satire. Instead, in the quasi-tradition sketched here, of men
writing about men nursing men, the ideal has been removed from childhood and from true mothering, even from women, and relocated in the
comradely world of men caring for men whose autonomy is respected and
whose space is not violated.[20] Despite suffering and death, war and social
oppression, these men will not betray their charges. Their care is unexpected, remarkable simply for existing. For other men they are safe and
known and not in bondage as women are to the betraying body.

What conclusions shall we draw from a powerful body of imaginative
literature that depicts men rather than women as the true caretakers? We
will not blame mothers. Mother-failure is inevitable, for mothers are human beings. In the present state of the world, mother-failure constitutes
an exile for men that is not quite so final for women. We may hold our
children, attempt to be better mothers. We may also choose to become

nurses. What seems needed is an acceptance of the possibility of care between human beings, a distinct, noninvasive care; and I suspect this possibility must exist outside the nursing profession before it will be credible (at least to those who are not ill) in its practitioners. Love and care and human contact must be open to men and to expression between men. We all have bodies. We all have lost the mother of our infancy no matter to what degree we had hoped to possess her. We all will die. If our society is to be free of antifeminism, men must begin to share the burden and pleasure, the joy and grief of caring physically for others with the other half of the human race.

Notes

1. Literary images constitute a special "reality." Insofar as every story, even the one told casually to a friend immediately after an event, differs from a transcript of that event, that difference is determined by the meaning or the sense of life to be conveyed, the teller's conscious and unconscious values. This shaping is what makes literature valuable in every society, and its analysis is one of the functions of literary criticism.

2. Leslie A. Fiedler, "Images of the Nurse in Fiction and Popular Culture," *Literature and Medicine* 2 (1983):79–90. Reprinted in this volume, chap. 4, pp. 100–112

3. I regard works in this body of "mainstream" literature as more or less equally accessible, constituting a literary "world" that has conditioned our perception of social and individual life—and that continues to do so. For this reason and because I am not tracing a historical development in literature but a cultural attitude that writers express whether or not they have read their predecessors, I have not discussed their works in chronological order.

4. Catherine Barkley in Hemingway's *A Farewell to Arms* (New York: Scribner's, 1929) is at first glance an exception, but one who suffers for her normality. She dies in childbirth, and her child dies too. The wartime fantasy ends without issue: ". . . but that was in another country;" run the lines that inspired him, from Christopher Marlowe's *The Jew of Malta,* "And, besides, the wench is dead" (Act 4, Scene 1, lines 41–42). See Carlos Baker, *Ernest Hemingway: A Life Story* (New York: Scribner's, 1969), 383.

5. Eric J. Cassell has described this alteration persuasively in *The Healer's Art* (New York: Penguin, 1976).

6. Nancy Chodorow, *The Reproduction of Mothering* (Berkeley: University of California Press, 1978).

7. Philip E. Slater, *The Glory of Hera: Greek Mythology and the Greek Family* (Boston: Beacon Press, 1971).

8. Lillian Smith's *Killers of the Dream* (New York: Norton, 1949) and James Baldwin's "Going to Meet the Man," in *Going to Meet the Man* (New York: Dial, 1965) are classic descriptions of this phenomenon. Both account for the part played by women, black and white, in the social paranoia of white men.

9. Nursing is to some degree the prisoner of the name given the profession. "Nurses" are, semantically, substitute mothers; they nurture and feed. See Claire Fagin and Donna Diers, "Nursing as Metaphor," *New England Journal of Medicine* 309 (14 July 1983):116–17.

10. Ken Kesey, *One Flew over the Cuckoo's Nest* (New York: New American Library/Signet, 1962), 30. All subsequent page references are to this edition and will be cited parenthetically in the text.

11. The Chief's return to sanity is signaled by his relinquishing this habit. The first hint is his seeing, as if for the first time, the landscape outside his window *as it is*. Near the end of the novel he is able to describe without reification how a scene appears at sunrise: "It looked at first like the leaves were hitting the fence and turning into birds and flying away" (p. 199).

12. Ann Douglas has described the historical grounds for this perception in *The Feminization of American Culture* (New York: Knopf, 1977).

13. Leo Tolstoy, *The Death of Ivan Ilych*, trans. Louise and Aylmer Maude, in *The Death of Ivan Ilych and Other Stories* (New York: New American Library/Signet, 1960), 136. All subsequent page references are to this edition and will be cited parenthetically in the text.

14. Walt Whitman, "The Wound-Dresser," lines 5–6, from *Leaves of Grass* (1891–92), in Walt Whitman, *Complete Poetry and Collected Prose*, ed. Justin Kaplan (New York: Library of America, 1982), 443. All subsequent line references are to this edition and will be cited parenthetically in the text.

15. Walt Whitman, "Vigil Strange I Kept on the Field One Night," lines 9–17, from *Leaves of Grass* (1891–92), in Walt Whitman, *Complete Poetry and Collected Prose*, ed. Justin Kaplan (New York: Library of America, 1982), 438–39. All subsequent line references are to this edition and will be cited parenthetically in the text.

16. Jorge Luis Borges, "Remorse for Any Death," line 7, trans. W. S. Merwin, in *Selected Poems, 1923–1967*, ed. Norman Thomas Di Giovanni (New York: Dell/Delta, 1979), 15.

17. George Gordon, Lord Byron, "Love and Death," lines 9–12, in *The Poetical Works of Byron*, Cambridge Edition, rev. ed., ed. Paul Elmer More (Boston: Houghton Mifflin, 1975), 206.

18. Hart Crane, "Episode of Hands," lines 8–15, in *The Complete Poems and Selected Letters and Prose of Hart Crane*, ed. Brom Weber (Garden City, N.Y.: Doubleday/Anchor, 1966), 141. All subsequent line references are to this edition and will be cited parenthetically in the text.

19. This proportion of satiric detail to violated ideal was established by Mary Claire Randolph, "The Structural Design of the Formal Verse Satire," *Philological Quarterly* 21 (October 1942): 368–84.

20. May Sarton's novel *As We Are Now* (New York: Norton, 1973) may be regarded as a woman's version of this pattern: the heroine is cared for—and taught by—a good woman nurse, and the lesbian reading is equally plausible, equally inadequate. Whether sufficient trust and lack of ambiguity are possible when patient and nurse are of opposite sex awaits the investigation of social scientists as well as writers of fiction.

Barbara Melosh

6. "A Special Relationship": Nurses and Patients in Twentieth-Century Short Stories*

Nurse characters appear in surprising profusion and various guises in fiction. In sympathetic portraits, they are nurturing mothers or caring allies. Sometimes the nurse is the emblem of the outsider, a pathetic spinster or strange recluse. In other depictions, nurses' authority and expertise set them beyond the bounds of proper female behavior: they are shown as icy martinets or sexual predators, threats to male prerogatives. Other stories reveal the nurse as an initiate into esoteric secrets: her knowledge of the body and her proximity to feared illness and death draw her closer to the worlds of forbidden sexuality, human frailty and evil, and supernatural horror. Represented in every genre—mystery, romance, science fiction, and horror—nurse characters have even claimed their own: thousands of young girls thrill to the adventures of Sue Barton and Cherry Ames, just as their adolescent and adult counterparts follow the troubled fortunes of protagonists in the ever-popular "nurse-romances." And nurses also occupy the canon of "high" literature: William Faulkner, Ernest Hemingway, Dorothy Parker, Ellen Glasgow, and F. Scott Fitzgerald, to name only a few, have all produced memorable nurse characters.

Nurses themselves have been close readers of, and sometimes contributors to, this literature. Professional journals, concerned with public image in their struggles to upgrade nurses' status, have consistently reviewed the depiction of nursing in literature, advertising, television, and film. At times the journals have included didactic short stories, using the vehicle

*I acknowledge with gratitude the helpful comments of Anne Hudson Jones and other participants in "Images of Nursing in History, Literature, and Art," a conference held at the Institute for the Medical Humanities, Galveston, Texas, November 1983.

of fiction to convey a model of proper professional behavior or to explore the conflicts and ethical dilemmas of work. Other nurses have written stories about their work as recruitment tracts, aiming to inspire young women to join the ranks. Whether as critics or writers, nurses have assumed that fiction reflects and in turn shapes public opinion; and they have worked vigorously to intervene in that process.

If literature is a form of ideology, as Marxists and feminists have argued—and I would agree—then such interventions are highly appropriate. Nonetheless, I would suggest that by insisting on a kind of socialist realism—a depiction of nursing that conveys an ideal version of the profession's goals and activities—nurses have overlooked some of the revelations that this fiction contains. Rather than viewing literature as a tarnished mirror, this reading approaches fiction as a metaphorical statement. A writer is more than a transparent eye or reflecting glass; the lens of fiction inevitably refracts and transforms. Nor is a short story or novel a Gallup poll. Fiction does not represent public opinion in any direct way; or if it does, judging from the wide diversity in depictions of nursing, then "the public" is a fragmented and divided entity indeed. Further, one might argue that the best fiction engages us by its originality more than through its ability to embody or restate widely held views; we turn to literature to find new connections, to see life freshly.[1] Can this kind of art, valuable for its unique perspective, lead us to greater understanding of the commonplace; from metaphors related to nursing to any useful insight about nursing itself?

In trying to make this leap from the created world to the world of experience, I would argue that the individual vision of fiction is inextricably connected to the larger social life in which its author is situated. Fiction that "works" does so, I think, because it brings us to a new way of seeing through the medium of commonly understood categories and associations. Good writers remake the language, tear down and reconstruct our assumptions, but they must begin with materials we know; the created world is rendered intelligible by its correspondences to the world of experience. To draw conclusions about social life or history from fiction, the critic must explicate the intricate mediations between these worlds. If fiction is constructed by a process of significant selection, then we can look behind its edifice to the scaffolding of common cultural materials: the structure of shared language, allusions, types, categories that constitutes the medium of communication between author and audience.

To share a common language is not to agree on everything that is said:

I use the linguistic analogy deliberately to avoid the assumption of underlying social consensus sometimes made in this kind of criticism. Nor is this set of associations fixed or immutable. Like language itself, the content and meanings of metaphors vary with time, setting, and audience. And, again as in linguistic communities, the audience at any given moment constantly introduces its own variations: readers bring new meanings to the text by resisting, reinterpreting, or even simply misunderstanding what is said.

Taking the measure of the created world, the critic necessarily compares it with the world of experience, but not as a way to hold fiction to a literal accounting. The distance between observed reality and the truth of fiction, far from disqualifying it, constitutes the main strength and interest of fiction. These transformations are keys to the cultural ideology that shapes both fiction and social life. Because short stories operate under strict constraints of compression—every detail and image must count—they are especially well suited to this kind of analysis. More varied and complex than genre literature or didactic stories, and for the most part more self-conscious in its use of character and imagery, short fiction provides a revealing index of the cultural meanings that surround and interpret nursing. In analyzing these stories, I have focused on the question of artistic selection: why have these authors chosen to portray nurses? What images, characteristics, and emotions do the writers associate with their nurse characters? What would readers have to know about nurses to make the characters intelligible? What would they have to believe to make the portrayals convincing? And finally, what place do nurses occupy in the moral universe of the fictions?

I identified short stories with nurse characters by using the *Short Story Index,* a bibliographic aid to short fiction organized by subject.[2] The subject guide appears very thorough: a number of the stories listed under "Nurses and Nursing" contained only incidental nurse-characters. The *Index* itself is quite selective, though, since it includes only stories that have appeared in anthologies. Therefore, it cannot be taken as a reliable source for the presentation of nurses in mass market magazines or as documenting popular fiction more generally. Nonetheless, the *Index* does offer the advantage of a heterogeneous sample because anthologies themselves are directed to a variety of different audiences and compiled for different purposes. The fiction indexed here leans toward "high" literature on the one hand—stories that are reprinted for their special literary merit, often in "prize" anthologies, or published in collections of a single author's work.

On the other hand, the *Index* also picks up genre anthologies, collections directed to afficionados of mystery, horror, science fiction, or, in several examples, nurse stories themselves!

I selected the fifteen stories examined in this essay from fiction listed in the *Short Story Index* from 1900 to 1981.[3] I eliminated stories published before 1900, those in translation, and listings repeated from one volume to the next. I also omitted didactic stories directed to young women, the so-called teen-age nurse stories; I have discussed this genre elsewhere.[4] Of the approximately 144 stories that remained, I have read 58, a selection largely determined by what was available to me. In the considerable variety of genre and intention that these stories represent, the two most common subjects are nurses' relationships with patients—both working and sexual relationships—and nurses' romantic and sexual encounters with partners who are not patients. The depictions of love and sex often evoke associations with the work of nursing; however, I chose to focus on stories of nurses and patients because these more often portray nurses on the job.

Prurient, comic, dramatic, sentimental, or grotesque, the stories vary widely in tone but are related by their use of three recurring themes: power and inequality between nurse and patient; the test posed by illness or impending death; and the costs and rewards of empathy. The unusual circumstances of illness work as a literary device to allow searching into character or to explore relationships that transgress the boundaries of normal social behavior. In this realm, characters exercise sexual license; regress to childlike behavior; attain mystical or supernatural perception. Sometimes nurses are guides on these excursions; sometimes they are simply the objects of their patients' disturbed fantasies. But in all they are seen as insiders, initiates into a domain of powerful emotion and uncommon experience.

Power and Inequality: The Theme of Sexual Inversion

In stories of male patients and female nurses, the most common fictional pairing, writers often play on the inverted sex roles of helpless patient and powerful nurse. Stripped of accustomed privileges of race, gender, and class by illness, male patients find themselves dependent on women in stories that explore psychological complexities of power and inequality through this inversion.

In "A Drink of Water" (1956), T. K. Brown, III, develops this theme in a lurid story of a badly wounded man, left blind and limbless after he trips a concealed mine in World War II Palermo.[5] As Fred MacCann regains consciousness and realizes his condition, he sinks into despair. His gentle nurse Alice gradually draws him back to life. Dependent on her for all his physical care and much of his information about the world, Fred relives the infant's fusion with its mother. In images of regression, the author evokes this psychological state: he emerges from "the womb of his defensive obsession" (p. 181); finds himself lying "in some sort of crib" (p. 182); and finally becomes "a child again under the impact of such anguish" (p. 183). Once a lusty, athletic man, Fred now confesses his childlike dependency to Alice, who accedes laughingly, "I am your will. . . . You are my baby" (p. 186).

The ominous undertones in this unbalanced relationship foreshadow the plot's next twists. First, Alice shatters the comfort of Fred's infantile regression. Proclaiming that "I am another person, too. . . . I am a woman" (p. 189), she caresses his body in an unmistakable sexual initiative. For an uneasy moment, Fred feels betrayed and mocked, but then he exults in his reclaimed sexuality. Soon, though, his unease returns. One day Alice calls him her "man thing," (p. 198), and confides what he has begun to fear: she hates men. His stomach turns as she lavishes kisses on him, for he now realizes that she loves him only as "a phallus on its small pedestal of flesh. Not planted anywhere, not sacred in any way, by no means inviolable: any woman could carry it off and use it" (p. 199). Devastated by her betrayal, he kills himself.

Jack Dann's "Camps" (1979) uses the same themes of sexual regression and obsession.[6] In this science fantasy story, sickness opens another realm of experience as the critically ill Stephen "enters pain's cold regions as an explorer . . ." (p. 101). Told from the viewpoint of this feverish patient, the story records his confused images of his nurses. Sometimes they appear as the imagined projections of Stephen's disordered state; at more lucid moments, Stephen's descriptions seem reliable. An early comparison of his day and night nurses suggests his regression to infantile fantasy of the mother. His sympathetic day nurse is the "good" mother, giving and nourishing; his dour night nurse is the "bad" mother, withholding his Demerol and denying his requests for soothing ice. Josie, the day nurse, is all women—"Stephen is reminded of old women and college girls" (p. 102); she is also one woman, recorded in another of Stephen's observations as "not a pretty woman—too fat" (p. 109), with a "musky odor" (p. 102), her face "prematurely lined" (p. 105), "an overly full mouth," and breasts too small for her body (p. 109). An aura of ambiguous and forbidden sexuality surrounds the nurse character, who seems at once too sexual for a mother and too matronly for a lover. But even as Stephen registers her flaws, his desire grows into obsession. Josie's response mirrors her body's ambiguous promise. On the one hand, she gently deflects his declarations of love, long inured to the transference and regression of very sick patients. When he begins to recover, she turns her gaze from his naked body. When he teases her for this new reticence, she explains, "When you were very sick, I washed you in bed as if you were a baby. Now it's different" (p. 114). On the other hand, in scenes that seem to be more than Stephen's fantasy, she embraces him. Even as she murmurs, "This is wrong," they kiss and he "feels her thick tongue in his mouth . . ." (p. 115).

Meanwhile, Stephen slips in and out of terrifying nightmares of a Nazi death camp. He mumbles German in his sleep, though he does not know the language. As he tells Josie his dreams, she recognizes authentic detail from her own life; she was one of the first nurses to enter the camps with the Allied Forces. Through the mystical bond of his dependence, Stephen has become trapped in her past and must live out the nightmare in order to get well. In a terrifying climax to his series of nightmares, Stephen dreams of escaping execution by hiding in a mass grave: only then does he recover from his illness in waking life. But still he clings to Josie, bound by her care and the compelling intensity of the nightmares. Like a child, he cries, "I don't want to leave, I want to stay with you." Like a good mother, she firmly turns him out into the world: "Stop that talk, you've got a whole life ahead of you" (p. 125).

Set in a Harvard infirmary, John Bovey's "Famous Trials" (1980) evokes the same sense of estrangement as the sick male student slides into the esoteric world of illness.[7] The strange smells and forbidding appearance of the infirmary mark it off from the rest of the university. Exchanging his own clothes for institutional apparel, he undergoes a rite of passage. The anonymous hospital robe, "bleached almost to transparency" (p. 138), is a symbol of identity blurred and diminished. Yet, although he is uneasy in this unknown world, the weary student also welcomes the chance to retreat to it: He "pushed [his] way into this cocoon" (p. 138).

As in Dann's story, the image of regression is heightened by the day and night nurses, again the "good" and "bad" mothers of infantile fantasy. The disapproving night nurse, "whose mouth often puckered all around as though drawn by a cord," will not let him out of bed, forcing him to use a bedpan (p. 139). Her controlling behavior accentuates his loss of adult status, the "unmanning" of illness. In a reinforcing image, the narrator confesses that even when the day nurse lets him walk to the bathroom, he is "too weak to piss standing" (p. 140). Amelie Corrivau, the day nurse, is ethereally beautiful, with "shining, reddish hair," "enigmatic" smile, and "faintly exotic" accent (p. 138).

In the inverted world of the hospital, sex stands for death: no longer opposing forces, Eros and Thanatos are linked. As his ordinary life recedes into the absorbing world of the infirmary, the narrator is gripped with desire for Amelie: "Her touch caused a turmoil in [his] blood" (p. 141). Male sexuality, usually shown as active or aggressive, is here rendered in passive images, a language of helpless desire that suggests both allure and danger. The implied threat of this languid world becomes clearer as the patient probes the secret of a closed door. In that room, he discovers, a Harvard student recently died. Still he sinks deeper into the seductive domain of illness. He takes a book from the dead student's room and tells Amelie, ". . . it's crazy: the longer I stay here, the less I care about getting out" (p. 143). The ease of the infirmary has become more compelling than the world of action; he languishes dreamily in a place where, as he muses, "There's nothing left for you to decide" (p. 144). A nightmare jolts him out of this engulfing passivity. He dreams of being dragged down into the underworld of easeful death, the only final place of refuge from will and choice.

The movement of the story reverses as the narrator prepares to leave the infirmary and reenter his old life. He goes back to the closed room to return the book and finds Amelie weeping as she mourns the dead student. Comforting his nurse, he takes control of the relationship in which he was once as passive as an infant. He pulls off her cap, the emblem of her professional authority, and loosens her hair, described in an image of desire and hidden threat: ". . . so full and rich and yet coarse. The odor of violets floated into [his] nostrils" (p. 146). This time, though, he resists the allure and gets ready to go home. At his discharge, Amelie will not acknowledge the intimate moment they shared, and says goodbye to him with cheerful impersonality.

The story ends on an arresting image of double betrayal. Having discovered the truth of Amelie's world—that the infirmary is not a retreat but instead the place of final reckoning—the student escapes back into ordinary life. The young man vows to hold on to the dark knowledge of that room, "of pain and dying and loving without hope" (p. 149); and yet he also recognizes that he has turned from the hospital to the commonplace world where such truths seldom intrude. When Amelie says, "We'll miss you. . . . come back and see us" (p. 149), he is stung by the implication that he is no longer one of "*us,*" the intimates of the ward. In the last line of the story, he accepts the implied rebuke, and with it the bitter recognition of his own flight from pain: "But though I wrapped her words in forgiveness, my mouth was dry with a toxin for which there was no antidote" (p. 149).

These three stories all depend on the powerful emotions associated with sex and death, Eros and Thanatos. Brown's "A Drink of Water" manipulates the complex psychological associations surrounding women as both objects of desire and threats to autonomy. In her maternal care of Fred, the nurse seems to nurture Fred only to end by devouring him. As his lover, she seems to affirm his adult status and his separate identity, but later we see her literally incorporating him, taking over his body. In this revealing document of fifties' misogyny, the author speaks through his protagonist: we are meant to feel, through Fred's experience, the destructive power of unleashed female sexuality. Brown risks losing his audience with the luridness of his plot and characterization. Fred's injury is so severe, his nurse so peculiar, that readers may have trouble suspending disbelief to enter the fictional world. Yet in 1958, the story won an O. Henry award; and even for this skeptical feminist reader in the 1980s, the story holds a kind of fascination. Brown successfully exploits the raw emotion—pity, revulsion, and most of all fear—evoked by Fred's terrible helplessness. Self-consciously linking this dependence with the experience of infancy, Brown makes Fred the embodiment of deeply held fears of women. In this nightmare vision, the controlling mother of infantile fantasy is made real; and just as an American man in the fifties might expect, she appropriates his penis.[8]

Dann's "Camps" and Bovey's "Famous Trials" filter these emotions and associations through a more critical perspective. Even as we are drawn into the feverish perceptions of both sick patients, we are also reminded that they may not be wholly reliable narrators. Indeed, the stories engage the reader with this ambiguity: we puzzle over what is fantasy or projection, what is real. At first, the nurses seem to occupy the grounded and material world of ordinary life, and their professional distance heightens the reader's sense of the distorted perceptions of their patients. But then Dann and Bovey introduce plot twists that lead us to reassess the patients' reliability, raising new doubts about the line between fantasy and reality. At critical points in both stories, the nurse characters respond to their patients' sexual overtures. In these fleeting moments, the nurses are not just projections of male desire, but in fact sexually available. In Dann's supernatural story, the infantile fantasy of fusion with the mother becomes horribly real. Caught in a nightmare world, the patient is condemned to relive his nurse's history. In both stories, the nurses at first appear as the other-worldly creatures of their patients' fevered imaginations; by the conclusions, they are revealed as truly otherworldly, inhabitants of a realm of secrets and painful truths. As women and as nurses, they are the other—initiates into special knowledge that is both feared and desired. They are emblems of the unconscious, representing the inner struggle between the life force and the will to die. And these stories work, I think, because in our culture ambivalence about women is so powerful that female nurses can effectively stand for the profound fear and longing associated with both sex and death.

The many reworkings of this theme of sexual inversion suggest its fundamental appeal. In stories like Brown's, the nurse-patient relationship is a device for reexamining the battle of the sexes: the authors focus on men's efforts to reclaim their dominance. Brendan Gill's "And Holy Ghost" and William Kotzwinkle's "Stroke of Good Luck: A True Nurse Romance" both show the nurse-patient relationship as a challenge to male control.

Brendan Gill's "And Holy Ghost" (1945) portrays the power struggle between a manipulative male patient, Rocco, and his nurse, a young nun.[9] They are about the same age, but as she reflects, "He was twenty, but he was also six. As she was twenty-five, but also eighty" (p. 211). The shifting viewpoint shows both sides of the struggle. She is attracted to him in spite of herself, a response she tries to sublimate and justify in an earnest effort to convert him to Catholicism, the church of his Italian background. She recognizes that her attention to him exceeds her professional obligations: "Sooner or later, these [special favors] would be matters for confession" (p. 211). Her feelings toward him are both maternal and sexual; exasperated with him, she thinks to herself, "She could spank his round, hard bottom" (p. 211). The story's shifting point of view shows Rocco's scheming for her attention. Attracted to a nun, he responds to her both as the ideal woman and the emblem of forbidden sexuality, comparing her quiet strength to the strident demands of his female relatives, "the harpy voices he had lived with all his life . . ." (p. 220). He asks for the priest, raising Sister Louise's hopes for his salvation. But the jaded priest is not convinced that Rocco has made the sincere confession of faith that must precede adult baptism. Rocco finally persuades the nurse to baptize him instead. The baptism represents Rocco's triumph in the struggle of wills, a form of sexual conquest. He has overcome the nun's misgivings yet still withheld his soul: the last line of the story reveals that he is still an unbeliever. And yet what has he won? The ending maintains the ambiguity of this nurse-patient relationship. As Sister Louise stands and sprinkles the supine Rocco, the baptism itself becomes an image of sexual inversion. Rocco's triumph has come through acquiescence, not the usual route for men. Sister Louise has bent to his will, in one sense, but she has also bound him to her church.

William Kotzwinkle's "Stroke of Good Luck: A True Nurse Romance" (1971) is a tongue-in-cheek version of the time-worn stock "plot" of pornography, the delights of mining the sexual promise of the knowing nurse. A fourteen-year-old boy, hospitalized for an appendectomy, lusts after the pretty nurse who shaves his body and seems to touch him provocatively. After his surgery and discharge, he goes to his physician's office where the doctor orders a follow-up sperm test. The accommodating office nurse then collects the specimen with an alacrity that exceeds the usual boundaries of professional commitment, a procedure recorded in several pages of closely observed, if not exactly clinical, detail. The story ends as the adolescent narrator exults in his unexpected sexual initiation, the "stroke of good luck" that accompanied his illness.

The battle of the sexes is a subject hardly restricted to stories about nurses, of course; it appears over and over again in our imaginative literature. Like countless other writers, Gill and Kotzwinkle use the war between men and women as the dramatic conflict that animates their stories. Nurse characters and hospital settings are deliberate selections that bring heightened emotion to a frequently explored subject. The inversion of sexual prerogatives engages the reader anew, changing the terms and possible outcomes of the conflict. In Gill's "And Holy Ghost," the confident man is reduced to helplessness; the docile nun controls him. Kotzwinkle's "Stroke of Good Luck" plays on the ambiguous intimacy of the nurse-patient relationship. The adolescent patient feels initially controlled by the hospital nurse's touch; later, in a more confident moment, he can experience physical intimacy as a service relationship that he controls.

As these diverse examples show, fictional depictions of nurses repeatedly involve themes of sexual inversion and conflict. Some stories use the asymmetrical nurse-patient relationship to heighten our sense of the losses of illness: men relinquish their powers to women. Others focus on the psychology of dependence, exploring parallels between nurse-patient and mother-child relationships. Some take the psychological theme further, creating nurses who represent Eros and Thanatos. And still others use the relationship as an effective vehicle for more conventional plots; their nurses and patients are men and women who approach and retreat from one another in a situation charged with forbidden sexuality.

The Test of Illness

In contrast, two stories use the nurse-patient relationship as a literary device to reveal the character of the male protagonist. In James Hopper's "When It Happens" and Frank Tuohy's "A Special Relationship," the authors use the protagonists' illusions about their nurses to unfold the truth about these characters' lives. Through the experience of illness, these men teeter on the verge of self-knowledge. The stories subtly capture the quiet drama of decisive moments in individual lives. Both end with a sense of loss or missed opportunities; both men retreat before the challenges that these moments pose.

Hopper's "When It Happens" (1927) works with the cliché of the patient smitten with his nurse.[10] The narrator, a writer, recounts his old friend Sam Nolan's story of a recent hospital stay. In the telling, Sam repeatedly denies that he has fallen in love with his young private nurse, Marjorie Downe. Instead, he keeps insisting, he is only providing ideas for his writer friend by explaining "how it happens when it does happen" (p. 168). Sam is both protected and protector in the relationship; he is grateful for his nurse's efficiency and also moved by what he perceives as her youthful vulnerability. He describes her manner as "Childish and innocent. It—well, it drew the heart" (p. 163). He explains the compelling languor of the hospital to his friend: "I wanted to remain just as I was up there in my little room. Alone in that small, clean, white, quiet world built around me by Marjorie Downe [his nurse]" (p. 165).

Sam tells the story to try to explain away this experience, struggling to interpret his desire to escape as part of his illness rather than as an authentic response to his life. The narrator supplies this perspective on Sam's account by reflecting on his friend's "terrible wife" and his squandered talents. To please his acquisitive spouse, Sam builds tract houses instead of committing himself to serious architecture. At one brief moment in the story, he does flare into rebellion. When his domineering wife invades the peace of his hospital room with imperious demands for a new home, the usually docile Sam refuses. But almost immediately he backs down again. Giving up the possibility of escape and renewal, he dismisses Marjorie, returns to the ward, and soon after leaves the hospital altogether. Apparently resigned to his lot, Sam still feels the tug of a lingering disquiet.

The story works through its artful juxtaposition of two points of view: the writer-narrator, who sees Sam's trapped life and unrewarding marriage for what they are, and Sam, whose story discloses a man poised on the brink of a truth he refuses to confront. We never see the real nurse behind the protagonist's idealized vision. Instead, Hopper reveals the infatuation as Sam's wistful longing for lost innocence, his regret for the unrealized possibilities of his own youth.

Similarly, Tuohy's "A Special Relationship" (1969 or 1970) deftly contrasts the penetrating clarity of illness with the compromises and evasions of everyday life.[11] The story opens after Roland is discharged from the hospital. Grateful to his nurses, he sends chocolates to the staff and invites Sister Grainger to dinner and theater to acknowledge her special support during his illness. As their awkward evening unfolds, we learn through Roland's inner monologue what the hospital initiation has meant to him. A London art dealer, Roland had elected nonetheless to enter the hospital as a National Health Service patient. By using the state-supported care instead of a private physician, he is able to purchase a valuable La Tour painting. Among working-class people in the hospital, Roland is ashamed of his privileged life and anxious to win acceptance on the democratic terms of the ward, where class differences are leveled by illness and patients judge one another by the standards of manliness under pressure. When his colleague Adrian arrives with "embarrassingly expensive" fruit, Roland feels "exposed and condemned, as though he could never re-enlist in the comity of the Ward" (p. 112). But that night, one of the ward patients dies. The petty divisions of the outside world disappear again; faced with their own mortality, the patients unite in strong, unspoken camaraderie. Back in his tasteful flat, Roland feels "unutterably changed" (p. 110), restless and discontented with his old routine. By inviting Sister Grainger there, he is trying to recover the sense of purpose and clarity of the hospital, groping for some integration of its revelation into his ordinary life.

Instead, his evening with the nurse marks his final separation from the world of the ward. In unerringly selected detail, Tuohy sketches Roland's dismayed recognition that the nurse is not his equal. "Deprived" of her starched uniform and bereft of the authority of the ward, she is out of place, even intimidated in his flat (pp. 101–3). An initiate in the hospital, she is "like . . . a large and appreciative schoolgirl . . ." (p. 105) in his stylish realm. Inured to the strong emotion and physical realities of sickness and death, the nurse is nonetheless shocked at the frank language of the play. Embarrassed by her clothes, bored by her conversation, Roland sees Sister Grainger as his class and intellectual inferior even as he is chagrined by his own snobbery. Miserably he considers his "patronizing" invitation, the carefully cultivated taste of his flat, his name-dropping at the theater: "He had always suspected himself to be an awful little man; surely the case was proved" (p. 107).

These lines signal the double meaning of Roland's judgment that the nurse is not his equal, for the story both undercuts and confirms his initial respect for her. Naive about art and taste, she still understands the deeper truths better than he, and faces them resolutely. Tuohy explicitly contrasts the fabricated drama of the play with the other "theatre" (operating room) whose authentic drama is Sister Grainger's milieu (p. 105). During the evening she quietly tells him of her brief marriage to a private-duty patient, her own failed effort to remake her life. But she discovered that the special relationship of nurse and patient cannot transcend the realities of class differences. She recognizes, "He should never have married me," and concludes prophetically, "People don't change much, do they? It's no use pretending they do" (p. 112). Roland realizes that he too will fail to transform himself. When she leaves, he again regards his surroundings with pleasure, relinquishing the challenge of the hospital and his resolution to live a new life. The story concludes with a poignant image of the nurse, again both "a little apart" and "inside," initiate into a world at once narrower and infinitely broader than the one Roland inhabits: ". . . the special relationship was at an end. She was already standing a little apart, a nursing sister under the stars and the bare branches, inside the order of things" (p. 114).

The Work of Caring

Other stories turn from the psychological meaning or social revelations of illness to consider the nurse-patient relationship from the caregiver's point of view. Nurse protagonists often provide an opportunity for authors to explore the costs and rewards of empathy. With a few exceptions, these stories offer sympathetic portraits of working nurses and show considerable insight into the emotional stresses of committed work.

Two stories depict nurses who are overly involved in their patients' lives. Ben Ames Williams's "The Nurse" (1926) is a condescending character sketch of an officious practical nurse, Millie, a middle-aged woman who lives through "her" babies and mourns the end of each case until a new infant comes into her care. Dorothy Parker's "Horsie" (1933), a more complex and critical view of the class relations between nurse and patient, bases its deft humor on the nurse's clumsy attempts to fit into the household of her wealthy young employers, where she cares for the spoiled wife after childbirth.[12] Both nurses are pathetic, bereft of romantic love, without children of their own, without the comforts of wealth and privacy, and without even the dignity of recognized skills—their employers treat them like servants. Condemned to these empty lives, Millie and Horsie lack even the resources of rebellious spirits; instead, they are content to live vicariously through their patients.

On the other end of the spectrum, two stories celebrate the rewards of committed nursing. Mary Ellen Chase's *The Plum Tree* (1949), a short novel, lovingly portrays a kindly middle-aged nurse who runs a residence for the elderly with her more jaded partner and companion. The story follows two days in her life as she orchestrates a tea party, working to bring a moment of joy to three difficult old women who will have to be transferred to a psychiatric facility. In "The Enchanted Nurse" (1953), William Goyen's first-person narrator, an old man, remembers his experience as a physiotherapist in England during World War II.[13] Describing the mending bones of men strung on frames, Goyen uses the metaphor of lace being woven on looms; the orthopedic ward is "a world of spider architecture" (p. 243). The narrator recollects the intensity of his relationship with one badly wounded young soldier; "this work was the only reality and it drew all things to it" (p. 252). In this lyrical affirmation, the nurse's commitment heals the caregiver as well as the patient through "this mysterious double action, this marvelous reciprocity, the way we human beings work upon each other" (p. 252).

Significantly, both stories use sexually symmetrical nurse-patient relationships. Davy, the female nurse in *The Plum Tree*, cares for patients who are also older women; Goyen's narrator remembers himself as a young man caring for a young soldier. Though both have intimations of homosexuality, the possible threat of this association is defused in images of domesticity and nurturance; the love in these stories is more caritas than eros. Davy and Angelina have lived and worked together for forty years. Their names suggest that they are like a heterosexual couple, and their domestic routines recall a comfortable marital intimacy. Goyen's story is much less direct in suggesting the nurse's sexuality; perhaps it seems present mainly because of the pervasive association of male nurses with homosexuality, or of tenderness with women. Nevertheless, the story does seem to play on this association; Goyen's narrator describes his case as "a work of love," immediately modifying the romantic associations of the phrase with the words, "the mark of a good nurse" (p. 252). The unusual choice of a male protagonist amplifies its celebration of commitment. The wartime setting evokes associations of the male camaraderie of battle. More, the uncommon expressiveness of a male narrator dramatizes the tenderness involved in good care. Stripped of more predictable and more ambivalent maternal and sexual associations, the image of nursing as "a work of love" takes on new life in both stories.

Two other stories of female nurses and female patients also focus on the empathy and intuition of nursing. In Ellen Glasgow's "The Shadowy Third" (1923; the slightly different original version was published in 1916), the nurse's sympathetic identification with her female patient is the pivotal element in this classic ghost story. The nurse initially accepts a difficult "mental case" because the patient is the wife of a charming and well-respected surgeon. Having assisted Dr. Maradick in the operating room and fallen under his spell, she is flattered when he requests her for the case. His wife is grief-stricken and apparently hallucinating in the wake of her daughter's death, her child by another marriage. Caring for the woman at home, the nurse begins to feel uneasy about the physician as she observes her gentle patient's fear and aversion toward her husband. Mrs. Maradick confides that the doctor has murdered her daughter to get the fortune left to the child by her father. The nurse weighs this information, unsure of her patient's mental stability. But she shares her patient's view of the world in a critical way, for she also sees the ghost of the dead child flitting through the house.

Meanwhile, the doctor prepares to rid himself of his wife and claim her inheritance. He gets the "alienist" (psychiatrist) on the case to commit Mrs. Maradick to an asylum. Nurse Randolph postpones this move once, but finally the day comes when Mrs. Maradick is taken away. As she leaves, the ghost child throws herself into her mother's arms, but only the nurse sees. To the alienist, also in the room, Mrs. Maradick's gestures are only another proof of her mental disorder. Soon the heartbroken mother dies in the asylum.

Fulfilling a promise to her, the nurse remains in the house with the ghost child, acting as Dr. Maradick's office nurse. The scheming physician, now the sole inheritor of the fortune, is preparing to marry again. Now that he is wealthy, his old girlfriend has accepted the proposal she once spurned. But the ghost child has her revenge at last. One night, as Dr. Maradick leaves the house to answer an emergency summons from the hospital, the nurse sees the child's jump-rope on the stairs. As she moves to light the hall, the physician trips on the rope and falls to his death.

Glasgow uses various facets of nursing to build the narrative and explain the protagonist's shifting sympathies. In the beginning we learn that Margaret Randolph is a recently graduated nurse, still not fully initiated into professional objectivity; she stands at the edge of the professional world. Her older mentor warns her about the cost of empathy, counseling her to think carefully before she takes on the mental case: "When you are drained of every bit of sympathy and enthusiasm, and have got nothing in return for it, not even thanks, you will understand why I try to keep you from wasting yourself."[14] The case forces her to weigh the claims of empathy and objectivity, imagination and scientific knowledge, spirit and flesh. As a woman, she is allied with the world of emotion and intuition, represented by the grieving mother and her ghost daughter. As a nurse, she belongs to the world of scientific knowledge, rational thought, and objectivity. At first infatuated with the surgeon and his mastery of the body, she is soon drawn into the female world of emotion and imagination instead. The character of the alienist further reinforces this division. Glasgow uses the early twentieth-century name for psychiatrist with ironic overtones. "Alienist" is a fit term for this doctor, chilly and remote, who views all human emotion as pathology. The nurse's female sensibility leads her to resist the doctors, even though she risks her future as a nurse by this rebellion. The ending affirms her intuition in a kind of feminist inversion of the plot in Brown's later "A Drink of Water." In "The Shadowy Third," a virtuous woman is revenged against a corrupt man; the traditional strengths attributed to female personality prevail over male aggression.

Nancy Hale's "Who Lived and Died Believing" (1942) explores the empathy between a female patient and her nurse by contrasting the patient's projections with the nurse's real situation.[15] The young nurse, Elizabeth Percy, worries over her emotionally disturbed patient, Mrs. Myles, while her boyfriend, Dave, a second-year medical student, grows impatient with her preoccupation. To Mrs. Myles, Elizabeth's relationship with Dave represents the possibility of love, "a flickering candle point upon the dark"

(p. 153). Elizabeth urges Dave to visit her patient, observing that Mrs. Myles responds to him; but he shrinks from this tortured soul. Gradually the patient improves, clinging to the hope that Elizabeth represents.

Meanwhile, in an ironic switch, the nurse comes to share a measure of her patient's disquiet. She knows that Mrs. Myles has broken down because her uncaring husband abandoned her when she was pregnant; shortly after, she miscarried. Elizabeth broods over her patient's unhappy situation, reflecting aloud to Dave, ". . . I keep thinking that's what love can do to you" (p. 155). She soon gains her own experience of the hazards of emotional commitment when she realizes that Dave does not love her and has no intention of marrying a lowly nurse.

At the end, Mrs. Myles finds out that Dave and Elizabeth have broken up and that her image of their secure love has been an illusion. Relinquishing her belief in an eternally sheltering love, Mrs. Myles completes her recovery. Together she and Elizabeth have lost their innocence but gained the strength to live without it. As the patient reflects to herself, "It was all gone, and love was gone too, and the candle flame had silently gone out. . . . It was all gone, and from now on the world was new, a page unwritten" (p. 165).

Finally, stories featuring nurse protagonists also record another side of caring: the strain, and sometimes the embitterment, of the nurse's repeated experiences of loss or failure. In the nightmarish "Old Soul" (1972), Steve Herbst comments on the cost of empathy for a young black nurse caring for a dying man. Attending him night after night, the nurse begins to feel submerged in his personality, experiencing a mystical knowledge of his past and future. The boundaries between the nurse and her patient blur; the cost of commitment is the erosion of self. Herbst's plot considers the fusion of infant and mother from the other side. If Dann's "Camps" and Brown's "A Drink of Water" dramatize the power of the mother, "Old Soul" portrays the adult's fear of the infant's voracious need. In his story, told from the nurse's point of view, we feel the caregiver's exhaustion and the emotional drain of a death watch.

A little-known story by F. Scott Fitzgerald, "An Alcoholic Case" (1937), effectively conveys another kind of strain—the frustration of patients who cannot be reached, the spectacle of lives wasted.[16] In this brief vignette, Fitzgerald captures the alcoholic's headlong self-destruction by observing him through the eyes of a determined young nurse. Grappling with her patient to keep him from the gin bottle, she resolves not to return to the case. Back at the registry, her supervisor offers to find a substitute. But the nurse decides that she will keep trying to save the alcoholic: "She was going to take care of him because nobody else would, and because the best people of her profession had been interested in taking care of the cases that nobody else wanted" (p. 320). In his room again, she dresses him and sees a copper plate in his chest, the result of a war wound. The nurse fights a sudden rush of sympathy, reminding herself that she must not yield to an emotion that will allow him to cajole liquor from her. But nothing can halt the alcoholic's inexorable ruin. A strange expression crosses his face, and, before her eyes, he dies. In the last lines, spoken by the young nurse to her supervisor, her own growing disillusionment echoes the alcoholic's nihilism: "It's not like anything you can beat—no matter how hard you try. . . . you can't really help them and it's so discouraging—it's all for nothing" (p. 322).

Conclusion

Surveying the variety of nurse characters in this sampling of short stories, what can we conclude about literary representations of nursing? These writers are not intent on making a statement about nurses and nursing; their stories cannot be read as direct commentaries. Instead, these short fictions take the relationship of nurse and patient as a revealing microcosm: a re-creation of the psychological dynamics of infancy; a skirmish in the battle of the sexes; or the setting for a moment of truth, a glimpse of the possibilities and limits of human relationships. Nonetheless, I think they do have special relevance for nurses, both for what they accomplish and for what they leave undone.

In the best of these stories, the authors' keen observations of the relationship of nurse and patient bring the pleasure of recognition that is part of our response to mimetic literature. We understand the seductive regression described in "Famous Trials"; we acknowledge the retreat from painful truths that occurs in Hopper's "When It Happens" and Tuohy's "A Special Relationship"; we share the frustration of the young nurse in "An Alcoholic Case." The clarity of insight in these stories, their psychological truths made palatable by the distance we gain through literature, can provide a real resource for nurses on the job as well as for the general readers to whom they are directed. Less familiar or less believable images can be instructive too. Nightmare visions, metaphors of impotence, and weird projections remind nurses of the strangeness of the hospital world and of their patients' fearful confrontations with mortality.

In another way, the significant omissions in these stories are also telling. Few of the fictions provide a sense of the complex technological and institutional workings of hospitals, possibly because of the limited compass of the short story: certainly there is an abundance of novels and nonfictional accounts of twentieth-century medical and nursing care, whether told from the inside view of practitioners or filtered through patients' accounts of illness. In the stories, even the most positive portrayals give little indication of the content and skill of nursing; little sense of nurses' relationships with medical and nursing colleagues; little idea of nurses' own lives outside hospital walls. To list these omissions is to point once again to the powerful salience of gender in nurse-patient relationships: repeatedly, fictional nurses are seen as mothers and lovers, whether divine or demonic.

How can nurses address this gendered and sexualized interpretation of their work? In protesting these depictions, as they have often done, nurses bring a valuable perspective to other readers. These challenges are themselves part of a movement for social change, an effort to make visible the selectivity of both artistic visions and cultural ideology itself. In turn, social change revises the materials and possibilities of imaginative literature. Over the twentieth century, both nurses' work and women's lives have changed dramatically, forcing some shifts in fiction. For example, I suspect that Williams's baby nurse and the pathetic Horsie are both less credible to readers today than they were in the 1920s and 1930s, and I find that Brown's story, written in 1956, already has the dated feeling of that era's especially intense sexual conflict. But the continuing re-creation of nurses as mothers and lovers attests to the durability of the tradition. To revise these deeply entrenched images will require more than skilled public relations. In the end, this literature inadvertently underlines the intertwined fates of nursing and the women's movement. As long as our culture sees women as other and lesser, nurses will be seen first as women and only secondarily as workers.

Notes

1. Genre literature is an exception: part of the pleasure of this form is its predictability or variation within strict constraints. For a good discussion of the

appeal and cultural meaning of genre literature, see John Cawelti, *Adventure, Mystery, and Romance: Formula Stories as Art and Popular Culture* (Chicago: University of Chicago Press, 1976).

2. Finding aids for novels about nurses are even more limited. The *Fiction Index* helps, though it ranges over many years and is highly selective, oriented toward helping public libraries select what to buy. But public libraries often keep older editions, and the source includes a detailed subject index and plot summaries. Genre literature about nurses is not indexed anywhere, as far as I know; you have to browse second-hand stores and become a presence at your local Salvation Army. Popular fiction about nurses is often reviewed in the columns of the *American Journal of Nursing* and *Public Health Nursing* (now *Nursing Outlook*). In addition to pointing toward portrayals of nursing in popular culture, these review sections also reveal contemporary professional responses to it. The bibliography in my dissertation, though far from complete, is probably the best place to start for a list of fiction dealing with nurses: see Barbara Melosh, "'Skilled Hands, Cool Heads, and Warm Hearts': Nurses and Nursing, 1920–1960," Brown University, Providence, R.I., American Civilization Program, 1979. My collection of fiction about nurses now belongs to the Nursing Archives, Mugar Library, Boston University.

3. Five of the stories I examine in this essay are available in *American Nurses in Fiction* (New York: Garland Press, 1984), a collection of nine stories that I have compiled and introduced. The five are T. K. Brown, III, "A Drink of Water"; Ellen Glasgow, "The Shadowy Third"; James Hopper, "When It Happens"; Dorothy Parker, "Horsie"; and Ben Ames Williams, "The Nurse." Other stories reprinted in the volume are Conrad Aiken, "Bring! Bring!"; Frederick Hazlitt Brennan, "Nurse's Choice"; Arthur Gordon, "Old Ironpuss"; and Ring Lardner, "Zone of Quiet."

4. For a discussion of genre literature about nurses, see Barbara Melosh, "Doctors, Patients, and 'Big Nurse': Work and Gender in the Postwar Hospital," in *Nursing History: New Perspectives, New Possibilities,* ed. Ellen Condliffe Lagemann (New York: Teachers College Press, 1983), 157–79.

5. T. K. Brown, III, "A Drink of Water," in *Prize Stories 1958: The O. Henry Awards,* ed. Paul Engle and Curt Harnack (Garden City, N.Y.: Doubleday, 1958), 179–201. All page references are to this edition and will be cited parenthetically in the text.

6. Jack Dann, "Camps," in *Timetipping* (Garden City, N.Y.: Doubleday, 1980), 101–25. All page references are to this edition and will be cited parenthetically in the text.

7. John Bovey, "Famous Trials," in *Desirable Aliens* (Urbana: University of Illinois Press, 1980), 137–49. All page references are to this edition and will be cited parenthetically in the text.

8. Interpreting this story in historical context, I have used Brown's "A Drink of Water" as evidence for the increasingly negative portrayal of nurses after World War II. As laypersons began to perceive nursing as skilled work and to associate it with prestigious and esoteric medical science, I argued, fic-

tional depictions of nursing expressed ambivalence and unease about women's fitness for the work. See Melosh, "Doctors, Patients, and 'Big Nurse.'"

9. Brendan Gill, "And Holy Ghost," in *Ways of Loving* (New York: Harcourt Brace Jovanovich, 1974), 208–21. All page references are to this edition and will be cited parenthetically in the text.

10. James Hopper, "When It Happens," in *The Best Short Stories of 1927*, ed. Edward J. O'Brien (New York: Dodd, Mead, 1927), 158–68. All page references are to this edition and will be cited parenthetically in the text.

11. Frank Tuohy, "A Special Relationship," in *Fingers in the Door and Other Stories* (New York: Scribner's, 1970), 101–14. All page references are to this edition and will be cited parenthetically in the text.

12. For an interpretation of this story as evidence for private-duty nurses' declining status in the 1920s, see Barbara Melosh, *"The Physician's Hand": Work Culture and Conflict in American Nursing* (Philadelphia: Temple University Press, 1982), 107–8, 191.

13. William Goyen, "The Enchanted Nurse," in *The Collected Stories of William Goyen* (Garden City, N.Y.: Doubleday, 1975), 240–54. All page references are to this edition and will be cited parenthetically in the text.

14. Ellen Glasgow, "The Shadowy Third," in *The Shadowy Third and Other Stories* (Garden City, N.Y.: Doubleday, Page, 1923), 5.

15. Nancy Hale, "Who Lived and Died Believing," in *The Best American Short Stories 1943*, ed. Martha Foley (Boston: Houghton Mifflin, 1943), 144–65. All page references are to this edition and will be cited parenthetically in the text.

16. F. Scott Fitzgerald, "An Alcoholic Case," in *The Bodley Head Scott Fitzgerald*, vol. 6, ed. Malcolm Cowley (London: Bodley Head, 1963), 314–22. All page references are to this edition and will be cited parenthetically in the text.

Bibliography

Bovey, John. "Famous Trials." In *Desirable Aliens*. Urbana: University of Illinois Press, 1980, pp. 137–49. Story first published in the *New England Review* in Spring 1980.

Brown, III, T. K. "A Drink of Water." In *Prize Stories 1958: The O. Henry Awards*. Edited by Paul Engle and Curt Harnack. Garden City, N.Y.: Doubleday, 1958, pp. 179–201. Story first published in *Esquire* in September 1956.

Chase, Mary Ellen. *The Plum Tree*. New York: Macmillan, 1949.

Dann, Jack. "Camps." In *Timetipping*. Garden City, N.Y.: Doubleday, 1980, pp. 101–25. Story first published in *The Magazine of Fantasy & Science Fiction* in May 1979.

Fitzgerald, F. Scott. "An Alcoholic Case." In *The Bodley Head Scott Fitzgerald*. Vol. 6. Edited by Malcolm Cowley. London: Bodley Head, 1963, pp. 314–22. Story first published in *Esquire* in February 1937.

Gill, Brendan. "And Holy Ghost." In *Ways of Loving*. New York: Harcourt Brace Jovanovich, 1974, pp. 208–21. Story first published in *The New Yorker* in 1945.

Glasgow, Ellen. "The Shadowy Third." In *The Shadowy Third and Other Stories.* Garden City, N.Y.: Doubleday, Page, 1923, pp. 3–43. Story first published in *Scribner's Magazine* in December 1916; the 1923 text contains some alterations from the original story.

Goyen, William. "The Enchanted Nurse." In *The Collected Stories of William Goyen.* Garden City, N.Y.: Doubleday, 1975, pp. 240–54. Story first published in *The Southwest Review* in 1953.

Hale, Nancy. "Who Lived and Died Believing." In *The Best American Short Stories 1943.* Edited by Martha Foley. Boston: Houghton Mifflin, 1943, pp. 144–65. Story first published in *Harper's Bazaar* in September 1942.

Herbst, Steve. "Old Soul." In *Orbit 11: An Anthology of New Stories.* Compiled and edited by Damon Knight. New York: Putnam's, 1972, pp. 169–75.

Hopper, James. "When It Happens." In *The Best Short Stories of 1927.* Edited by Edward J. O'Brien. New York: Dodd, Mead, 1927, pp. 158–68. Story first published in *Harper's Magazine* in May 1927.

Kotzwinkle, William. "Stroke of Good Luck: A True Nurse Romance." In *Elephant Bangs Train.* New York: Pantheon, 1971, pp. 98–107.

Parker, Dorothy. "Horsie." In *After Such Pleasures.* New York: Sun Dial Press, 1933, pp. 3–34. This collection of stories was adapted for the stage by Edward F. Gardner. His wife, Shirley Booth, played the leading roles for the production, which ran in New York for 23 performances. (See John Keats, *You Might As Well Live: The Life and Times of Dorothy Parker* [New York: Simon and Schuster, 1970], 187.)

Tuohy, Frank. "A Special Relationship." In *Fingers in the Door and Other Stories.* New York: Scribner's, 1970, pp. 101–14.

Williams, Ben Ames. "The Nurse." *Harper's Monthly Magazine* 152 (April 1926): 549–57.

Joanne Trautmann Banks

7. Votaries of Life: Patrick White's Round-the-Clock Nurses

The most practical book about nursing I know is not a text on physiology, an index of pharmacological effects, or a guide to the physical handling of bedridden patients. It is *The Eye of the Storm,* a six-hundred-page novel of decidedly highbrow mien by Nobel Laureate Patrick White.[1]

The journey into the core of this novel takes the reader through a terrain as vast as the mind's landscape and as formally complicated as the best of twentieth-century fiction. It is the same sort of journey one must take through, for instance, the novels of Marcel Proust or Virginia Woolf to arrive at a glimpse of timelessness suspended in daily life. One reward awaiting White's persevering traveler is nothing less than the transformation of nursing's daily chores—the bathing, the taking of vital signs, the response to a patient's call—into something entirely radiant. That transformation may be as close to the miraculous as many of us will get. Another reward is an infusion of new meaning into certain conventional images of nurses. In White, the mother, the seductress, the angel, and other images of nurses are *reaccepted* for the value at the bases of the stereotypes. The images are seen to have connections with primitive, and therefore inescapable, roles for women. They are mythic, finally, rather than stereotypic: not the mother who nurses and nags, but the Woman Who Gives You Birth; not the girl of easy virtue, but the Woman Who Makes Love to You; not the self-effacing martyr with no life of her own, but the Woman Who Eases the Passage into Death.

I call these matters practical on the grounds that the nurse who finds that daily work has joyful meaning is the same nurse who remains productive long after nursing's concepts and skills have become routine. In White's hands, moral insight is intensely practical.

But to convey that point, he must depend on a difficult combination of outright assertion, force of characterization, his and the reader's understanding of traditional women's roles, the circular patterning engendered by the change of shifts, and, withal, certain mysterious contiguities. Nor is it easy at first to follow the nursing theme in the novel. The reading I have given is wrested from the text and subtexts. At some stages, it may lie beyond White's original intentions for his book.

The novel is dominated, after all, not by nurses, but by one remarkable patient, about whom a few observations must be made. Elizabeth Hunter is a small woman of great age. As the result of a stroke, she can no longer independently feed or toilet herself. Often her thoughts are disconnected, as though the center cannot hold. She is, says one of the private-duty nurses who care for her at home, "a geriatric case approaching the expected conclusion" (p. 448). Only a few people attend her. She has outlived husband and friends, and she is not close, in the usual sense, to those who remain—namely, her middle-aged son and daughter and her attorney of many decades. These three are not even present very often. Therefore, by default, but also in some strange way by her design, Mrs. Hunter's most intimate relationships are with her two servants and, more important, with her nurses.

For one thing, the nurses come and go in predictable fashion every day. Every morning at 7:00 A.M. Nurse Badgery arrives (actually, "Sister Badgery," after the British-Australian fashion). She is followed by Sister Manhood at 3:00. Manhood, in turn, is succeeded at 11:00 P.M. by the night nurse, Sister de Santis. Here and there amidst the apparently major scenes of the novel they are glimpsed feeding their patient, sponging her, helping her to the commode. These minor activities add up. Nurse follows nurse, shift succeeds shift. Soon those twin professional banalities, duty and order, become the pins that hold together the novel's anatomy. The book's structure comes, very subtly, to rely on the reappearance of the next nurse.

First Shift: Sister Badgery and Authenticity

It seems to me that White begins with the assumption that the radiant and the profound in life are not very far from the daily and superficial. There are important humane and, finally, religious implications of that concept, about which I will need to say more later, but there are sarcastic aspects as well, residing chiefly in the first-shift nurse.

White has no shame when it comes to choosing names for his characters. Consequently, "Badgery" is a chiding, annoying, insinuating woman.

She talks too much, and in a trivially cheerful manner. Mrs. Hunter thinks her bossy; Mrs. Hunter's daughter calls her silly. Whenever the doctor is present—a man with whom she aligns herself in righteousness as over against the ignorant laity—she speaks to her patient in a voice of "exaggerated kindness" (p. 76). She "dear's" and "we's" Mrs. Hunter, and generally believes—this childless, middle-aged woman, who is at once skinny and melon-bellied—that her charge is a precocious toddler who does not always behave as she should.

There are social class issues at work behind the characterization of Badgery. That is, some of her qualities seem to derive from her social circumstances as much as from, say, a highly individualzed personality. It is not that White has prejudices for or against certain classes; in this book he sweeps through a wide variety of them without settling on any as a lens through which to view the others. It is just that he weighs class matters fairly heavily when he adds up the values of his characters, a habit of mind that is insightful with respect to the social class called private-duty nurse.

In the Hunter household, for instance, the nurses—including even de Santis, whose father was a doctor—have a status falling somewhere between their wealthy patient and the servants. But it is the servants with whom they share more daily, social characteristics. They eat with the housekeeper; they, especially Badgery and Manhood, behave naturally with her. The nurses carry out certain servantlike duties. They may even answer the front door and announce the visitors. Badgery seems to like these functions more than the other nurses, probably because she feels that by association with her wealthy patient or distinguished visitors, she increases her own worth: "She admired the rich, and enjoyed working for them because it gave her a sense of security, of connection, however vicarious" (p. 41). To increase that sense, she has taken to calling the midday meal "luncheon" in Mrs. Hunter's manner. And she is inordinately proud of having married a tea planter. Though she was widowed after a brief time—perhaps *because* of that convenient fact—she speaks of him in respectful tones. "My husband, Mr. Badgery, the tea planter," she says every chance she gets; "My husband was a tea planter, you know." She would be surprised to learn that Mrs. Hunter's foreign-titled daughter speaks of Badgery contemptuously as "the tea planter's widow" (p. 433). As a private-duty nurse whose patient is not ambulatory, Badgery has the run of a substantial house. Though this makes her feel the vicarious lady, she is in fact more in the position of a servant who manages a house while the lady is temporarily gone.

Her social status is further pinpointed by the fact that she speaks coarsely about money. Shortly after Mrs. Hunter's death, she thinks it perfectly appropriate to comment to her co-workers that she expected more than she got from the will and to speculate that the amount was dictated by someone other than Mrs. Hunter. Rather in the manner of a vulgar woman from a Restoration play, she says cheerfully that though five hundred dollars would enable her to take a bus tour to New Zealand—both islands, mind you—a larger legacy would have let her get as far as Japan. Her former patient has quickly been tidied into "such a generous woman—and lovely lady," and her only important remains into a few hundred dollars (p. 599).

Still, Badgery is not the thief that Mrs. Hunter's children think her and the other nurses. The son concludes: "Whatever their professional skill, nurses are renowned for being unpractical creatures, unless, as private nurses, they find themselves in a position to fleece their wealthier patients. Then some of them become most realistic. . . . where, for instance, does our mother's army of nurses *eat*?" (p. 264). And this from the daughter: "Are there any jewels left? . . . After the nurses have taken their pick?" (p. 584). But the children are wrong. White thinks Badgery vulgar and comic, but never immoral—unlike the children, one is inclined to add.

It is true that at times Sister Badgery's shallowness reaches almost criminal proportions, but always White turns it aside at the last moment into comedy. In that luncheon scene, for instance, soon after the death, Badgery fills almost all the silences left by the thoughtful, grieving de Santis and the housekeeper. Silence, says White, depresses Badgery. Her chattiness trivializes even intuition, a mode of knowing that White elsewhere ennobles as a part of the nurse-patient relationship. Badgery merely babbles boringly about her psychic powers: "I have my—*intuitions*. . . . In fact, if I wasn't a nurse—but I wouldn't give up nursing, not for worlds— I often think I might offer my services to the police. I am always right" (pp. 600–601). She never realizes how far from true knowing she is. Indeed her narcissism is remarkable. When de Santis mentions that her next patient is a girl whose legs are paralyzed, Badgery makes an attempt to imagine that plight, but just then the housekeeper puts a luscious dessert on the table and Badgery finds her "sympathy straying between her vision of this young girl and the slice of *Torte*. . . . 'Win Huxtable had a private case—a boy in an iron lung; it got her down in the end.' By which time Sister Badgery considered she might decently help herself to cream" (p. 601).

Strangely, using some of the standard criteria, Badgery is not a bad nurse at all. She is vigorous—"ostentatiously industrious," observes the attorney (p. 40)—and practical, the latter a quality required in a day nurse, according to de Santis. Things get accomplished in the light of day. At least they must be seen to be accomplished, and Badgery is suited to maintaining that busy illusion. She is the garrulous one who serves during the most sociable shift.

Indeed one begins to wonder if Badgery has any private self at all. Is she always "on"? Silence depresses her, and White never shows her, as he does the others, engaged in interior dialogue. What glimpses we do have of her thoughts are truncated. For instance, when she talks about psychic powers, she fears that she has revealed too much to a professional colleague. In other words, she is concerned only about her effect on her listeners; she never becomes her own audience.

In that respect Badgery helps to introduce one of the novel's most important themes: one might call it *authenticity*. The theme really belongs to Mrs. Hunter's son, who is a distinguished London actor—someone with the stature of a Richardson, Gielgud, or Olivier. But his mother's life illuminates it, and so do the nurses'. His mother had always been an actress. Whether she was using just the right tones to manipulate a dinner partner or making a grand entrance down the main staircase, Mrs. Hunter knew how to play to her fans. Even in advanced age, she consciously plays a certain role. When preparing for her son's long-awaited visit home, Mrs. Hunter has her sunken face made up in vivid colors and topped by a lavender wig. She wears an ancient silvery-rose gown and several rings. On making *his* entrance, her actor-son is rather thrown off his prepared lines by the sight of his fellow-actor, cast, he decides, as the Lilac Fairy. Recently, the son has played Lear to disappointing reviews. A good part of White's answers to the question of the true nature of the aging self is examined using *King Lear*'s images and values. The son learns, for instance, that Lear can be played "only by a gnarled, authentic man, as much a storm-tossed tree as flesh" (p. 350): not, in short, by a mere actor playing a part that fits him lightly.

The son and Sister de Santis see the two professions, acting and nursing, as sharing a concern with performance, in the sense of "how far to become involved" (p. 343) with the role one is playing. One wants, that is, to be a convincing Lear or private-duty nurse or whatever without being swept away by the emotions of the part, without losing that certain distance that is protected by technique. But then does one become mere technique, mere professionalism? Is nursing seen in this way a spurious profession with no genuineness to it? Must the actor-nurse give up the chance to interact authentically with other people?

These questions are answered, but not by Sister Badgery. When King Lear, his garments rent, has his famous vision on the heath, of human beings as "bare, forked animal[s]" (Act 3, Scene 4, line 116), he is not speaking of the likes of Badgery. She is never, as we have seen, without her role—her protective costume, as it were. Her visible costuming includes uniform, falsies, and interlock combs, but even when she changes into a street dress, she stays in role. Indeed, she has no lay self: "Sister Badgery, always at her most professional when out of uniform, gave him a therapeutic smile" (p. 575). When she goes on holiday, she travels as a nurse with other nurses.

Nursing—like acting, White gives us to understand—offers a useful route for those who would hide from their own humanity. In the face of madness, ills, and death, nursing can provide suitable methods for dehydrating one's emotions. Why Badgery chose this route, or if she chose it with deliberation, White does not say. In that respect he exploits her for his own ends. It is not that she is unintelligent; that much is fairly certain. She is only trivial. As a private-duty nurse, she can play the part of hanger-on to the wealthy. She is useful—as T. S. Eliot's Prufrock says in Shakespearean language—"To swell a progress, start a scene or two" ("The Love Song of J. Alfred Prufrock," line 113). But she is never herself even so much as the central character in her own play, whatever her narcissism. Probably, she likes neither her own body (she insists on absolute privacy when changing), nor the bodies of her patients. At best, she is indifferent to physicality. She compromises herself and her profession by preening for the doctor, any doctor, simply because he has what she sees as the right trappings. She married her husband for his position, and she is always more attracted to a person's technique than to his or her substance. Sister Badgery is known to be "a sucker for doctors, and tea planters, and actors' voices" (p. 562). The inauthenticity found in some brands of nursing is mirrored in her own tendencies.

Jessie Badgery is a happy woman. In her case, the unexamined life is a lark.

Second Shift: Sister Manhood and Human Love

On duty and off, Sister Manhood is lost in exploring the deep convolutions of the authenticity theme. Despite her sulky pretensions to adult freedoms, Manhood is in the full swing of late adolescence. For her, therefore, questions of personal identity are intense and choices about authenticity paramount.

In some ways Manhood is a nurse of the same stripe as Badgery. Superficially far different, they nonetheless share a tendency to bossiness, a quality pointedly withheld from the characterization of the third nurse. There is an element of Badgery too when Manhood finds it necessary to carry her "nursiness" into nonprofessional relationships. For instance, she makes some public health observations to her environment-polluting landlords to "prove [her] status from time to time" (p. 299). She has also adopted the professional's condescending pronoun and other terms of false endearment. Helping Mrs. Hunter onto the commode, Manhood chirps: "Say if we're not comfy, love" (p. 457). Moreover, she is perfectly capable of treating Mrs. Hunter like a child—though not precisely the same way Badgery does, and therein lies the beginning of certain subtle differences in the two nurses' adaptation of the professional relationship.

White depicts Badgery as a permanently childless woman, who exhibits, as a result, both sentimental and easily irritated attitudes toward childlike patients. In contrast, Manhood oozes with fecundity. In the tiny, withered person of Mrs. Hunter, Manhood comforts the baby she believes herself to be carrying at the time. White appears to look on this action as latently loving and dignified, especially as compared to Badgery's clucking maternalism. Even though Manhood is projecting onto that aging body the imagined body of a potential child of her own, she is at least acting out of her own authenticity if not in response to Mrs. Hunter's. And that is a step beyond Badgery.

Still, it is Manhood who is cast in the role of make-up woman and wardrobe mistress to the lead actress, Mrs. Hunter. When called upon, Manhood serves up her special training in these fields. Pulling out her palette of rouges and eyeshadows, her litter of wigs, her panoply of costumes, Manhood prepares Mrs. Hunter for the next curtain. The results are consistently grotesque. No one knows better than Sister Manhood just what the costuming hides—the cachectic body of a dying woman.

Thus her professional demeanor cracks from time to time, and the authentic—albeit immature—breaks through. From Cheerful Nurse she goes to Frightened, Angry Child. She uses phrases about Mrs. Hunter that Badgery, who is always in uniform, thinks thoroughly inappropriate. "The old bag" (p. 83), says Manhood, seeking to use language itself to fend off old people. Which of us, she wonders vulgarly, will find "the old thing" dead (p. 169)? (Answer: she will, because she needs to and deserves to.)

It is far harder for Manhood than for Badgery to achieve that competent impersonality that some believe is tantamount to nursing professionalism. At times Manhood is so detached that while sponging Mrs. Hunter she behaves as though she is peeling a fruit. But when she speaks of Mrs. Hunter as "a geriatric case approaching the expected conclusion" (for it was Manhood's description that was quoted earlier), she is striving to return to the assumed arrogance of her early training, as if adopting the professional approach of a Badgery could disguise her fear of being trapped by sympathy or horror. She is paid, she reminds herself, to perform certain duties, but not "suddenly to turn into a human being" (p. 105). But if she thinks to protect herself by repeating that patients are merely bodies, she is betrayed because, unlike Badgery, she looks honestly at bodies. She therefore sees that Mrs. Hunter's body is pathetic and, worse, the vehicle for very human vindictiveness, both of which qualities call forth "unprofessional" responses from her.

The struggle to maintain a sense of professional identity is all the harder because Manhood is a private-duty nurse. She does not have the supports of other personnel and institutional regulations—nor, for that matter, the alienation encouraged by unpleasant working conditions. Here in this large, well-staffed house, she is overfed and underworked. Here she meets the flirtatious son of her patient and learns all too much about Mrs. Hunter's family situation. How "[Manhood] wished it had been a hospital, when she could have produced a chart, handed over with efficient, completely impersonal cool, and swept off without further yakker" (p. 306).

Manhood is well aware of her predicament. She knows herself to be awash in confusion and hypocrisy. When she uses her "practised, nurse's voice" (p. 84) on Mrs. Hunter, while working off an internal image of her patient as a "rich bitch" (p. 310), she ends by loathing herself. Furthermore, she is "ashamed: she would have given anything to be gentle, serene, loving by nature" (p. 116). Off-duty, the struggle continues as she confronts, or rather does not confront, the men in her life. She thinks she is a "liar" and "cheat" (p. 530). In a frighteningly claustrophobic image for her depression, White writes: "Whichever way she looked she could see no end to her dishonesty: a vista of mirrors inside a mirror" (pp. 321–22).

Poor little Manhood. Nursing makes her unhappy, not so much because of any values inherent in the profession, but because it underscores the confusions in her personal life. Manhood cannot find authenticity in nursing because she has not yet resolved the ambivalences in her private life. The point is, Manhood cannot handle *human love*—that, in a sense, is the quest of the second shift—whether it offers itself in the guise of a patient or a lover and child. In this respect, the profession becomes a kind of laboratory in which the nurse investigates her capacity for love in any circumstance.

In Manhood's case, fear regularly gets in the way of love. For one thing, she has an insecurity bred in the bones of a provincial banana farmer's daughter who comes to the big city to study nursing and maybe catch a doctor for a husband. Manhood has spent a large part of her considerable courage in that act, for now, instead of relaxing into the satisfaction of her accomplishments, she evaluates her ignorance of books and theater and feels "for ever rooted in her origins" (p. 310). Her uniform does not hide her from herself. In fact, as a private-duty nurse, she meets patients and families whose proximal sophistication enlarges her fear. She does not really want a husband, after all, she thinks—not the famous actor, to whose bed she has entrée because she nurses his mother, nor the cultivated pharmacist, also met on the job, whose demonstrated knowledge of ideas and the arts enrages Manhood.

Moreover, just as she is determined to take her life into her own hands, this same pharmacist tries to pin her down into—to continue an earlier theme—a role for which she feels herself only an understudy and not yet ready to go on. The role is permanent Sexual Partner, which leads to Wife in the second act, and thereafter to Mother. This is where Manhood's deepest fear spreads itself, though again it is usually covered by anger.

Actually, Flora Manhood is well suited to any sensual role, fight it though she will at times. It is highly appropriate, for instance, that she loves to eat. When Manhood eats, she is engaged in one of life's primary pleasures. In contrast, Badgery, with whom she shares daily lunch, seems only greedy. Manhood loves good food, and she loves—this extremely pretty young creature—good sex, a fact that White everywhere advertises. He does not hesitate to dress her in a cerise-and-purple dress and pink plastic earrings. He intends the social message to read, "Desirable and Available," and he surrounds her with literate people. This "Flora" is in blossom, all right, and if "Manhood" does not immediately remind the reader of sexuality, White on one occasion causes the perspicacious Mrs. Hunter to think of her as "Sister Flora Pudenda" (p. 196).

Manhood wants the sexual experience, but not the dependence that she sees as its inevitable, claustrophobic accompaniment. At this stage of her struggle, in fact, she detests everything that reminds her of giving herself over to someone else. Unreasonably, she hates mutton chops because her pharmacist lover asks her to cook them so often. She is also revolted by them because they leave a residue of grease that she must wash off the plates: mutton fat as an image for semen.

In retreat from all this, Manhood thinks to move in with her female cousin, one "Snow" Tunks, who works as a bus conductor. With this character Patrick White is, in moral terms, his least attractive self. He creates in her a fat albino, whose lesbian love life is presented disgustingly amidst cheap alcohol, melting blue eyeshadow, and—interestingly enough—more mutton fat. Flora Manhood must flee again. Is sex everywhere, then, and everywhere horrible?

The trap is tightened for Manhood because she is pretty and a nurse, and therefore victimized by certain stereotypes about the profession. In a novel in which doctors are powerless beside the nurses, Mrs. Hunter's last doctor is especially pusillanimous in attempting to assert himself with Manhood—whose surname now takes on other overtones—by virtue of his professional *droit du seigneur*. When called to declare Mrs. Hunter dead, he first announces that their patient has "bought it all right" (p. 564) and then that Manhood now stands to receive some money from the will. Finally, as Manhood leans over the body to wash it, he thrusts at her from behind. The nurse pushes him off, claiming respect for her patient, only to hear the doctor reply disdainfully: "All the right sentiments! Like in the textbook. But don't you know a textbook is never for real?" (p. 565).

What is for real, then, about caring relationships? Manhood will not learn the answer through her one-night stand with Mrs. Hunter's son, to whom White assigns almost every positive and negative cliché one has heard about nurses, including that they are all sexually "corrupt" (p. 320). Postcoitally, he slips fast into the fantasy of marrying Manhood because, as everyone knows, nurses look after you at home and can go out to work if necessary. He turns to Flora's breasts as if to the consummate mother, an act that completes Flora's own fantasy.

Though it, too, is an ambivalent and possibly claustrophobic state, motherhood is the only role that may justify her existence, she thinks, and wipe out the fear that she has been promiscuous. Perhaps if she can produce flesh of her flesh, she can feed her hunger for love without simultaneously engendering that sense of separateness that presumes the possibility that one person can be over against another. Perhaps she will no longer be adrift. But Manhood does not become pregnant in the encounter with Mrs. Hunter's son. In White's universe, life does not beget itself in quite this manner; nor will closeness with Mrs. Hunter be achieved in this indirect way.

For it all returns to Mrs. Hunter. Manhood is her favorite—not because she makes up Mrs. Hunter's face, as the lawyer concludes, but because of the nurse's youthful sensuality. From Mrs. Hunter's perspective, we learn that "an animal presence is something the mind craves the farther the body shrivels into skin and bone" (p. 85). When she conveys this thought to Manhood, the nurse is, naturally enough, mightily offended to be labeled "the breeder" (p. 445), or to be told you can always tell by the smell when the she-goat has been to the he-goat. You will marry your pharmacist, Mrs. Hunter informs Manhood, giving her a ring to mark the engagement. With what agonizing fury does Manhood now twist in the trap.

"Do you love me, Nurse?" Mrs. Hunter asks on another occasion (p. 458), to which Manhood replies, unthinkingly, in conventional language: "What a thing to ask! Of course I love you. We all love you" (p. 458). But Mrs. Hunter has asked her question to ascertain whether Manhood would be willing to provide enough sleeping pills for a suicide attempt. Again, Manhood responds conventionally, and again Mrs. Hunter breaks through it: "Love is above ethics" (p. 459). Manhood feels she is being trapped and used in her work just as in her private life. The flirtatious Mrs. Hunter and Manhood's lover are conspiring against her.

Love—not conventionally expressed love—but deep connectedness: that is what simultaneously draws and repels Manhood. And somehow that fact is known to her patient. At a time when Manhood is struggling into full adulthood, Mrs. Hunter, though aging and disintegrating, is a guide: "Probably she [Manhood] felt contempt for everyone she knew, except perhaps Mrs Hunter: why not Mrs Hunter, when half the time she hated the old thing, she had not yet been able to decide" (pp. 176–77).

But she gets glimpses. There are times when something passes between Manhood and her patient that illuminates the common terms *empathy* and *compassion,* and simultaneously enlarges them far beyond textbook banalities. These are moments of deep human connectedness, but they arise out of commonplaces in nursing care. For instance, Manhood's and Mrs. Hunter's shared interest in make-up brings them together and allows their emotions to be sent back and forth as if on an electric wire. Or the sudden vision might descend during a backrub. Then, Manhood thinks, she gets past pitying to liking, "to almost having a love affair, the two of you and a sponge" (p. 105). On rare occasions, young Manhood is transformed from a brazen nonbeliever, convinced of life's emptiness, into a worshiper of what Mrs. Hunter represents: "Momentarily at least this fright of an idol became the goddess hidden inside: of life, which you longed for, but hadn't yet dared embrace; of beauty such as you imagined, but had so far failed to grasp . . . ; and finally, of death, which hadn't concerned you, except as something to be tidied away, till now you were faced with the vision of it" (p. 121). Always Mrs. Hunter's capacity for being cruel and manipulative returns to end the trance, but it works its magic on Manhood all the same.

Mrs. Hunter dies during Manhood's shift. It must happen then. Badgery would not have noticed it much; de Santis, as will be seen, has gone beyond its concreteness. Manhood needs to confront the end of human connection just when part of her has been given importantly to it. She responds at first with professionally distanced competence. She knows what to do with a body. But the struggling young woman in Nurse Manhood cannot hide her awe and her longing: "Though the mind can become as functional as the digestive tract after your feelings have been minced up fine, it did not prevent her touching the body several times when she had laid it on the bed, not expecting evidence of life (she was too experienced for that) but illumination? that her emptiness, she ventured to hope, might be filled with understanding" (p. 552).

Sensing that she must not run away completely into nursing professionalism lest she lose a precious chance, Manhood tries to learn tenderness through the experience of washing her first dead body. The task is terribly hard for her, armored as she is against the gentler feelings, but eventually "a kind of love began to jerk rather than flow along her straining arms" (p. 565). She waits then for Sister de Santis to come on duty in order to reestablish the nursely continuity, for which she now yearns. Together the two continue to prepare the body. And here, at least, Manhood is comforted. White draws a picture of the two nurses—quiet, practical, solicitous of one another—engaged in the traditional womanly task of preparing the dead for burial. As they work, their bodies—normally at a very professional distance from one another—bump, rub, and touch in a nearly balletic variant of an earlier scene with Snow Tunks and her lesbian roommate. It is then that Sister Manhood comes "closest to expressing the love she might have been too abashed to feel for Elizabeth Hunter" (p. 566).

The vision ends at this point. The death, the rituals, and the intimacies with her patient and her colleague are over. The shift has been completed, and Sister Manhood is released into the city at night. Now White's prose must run to stream of consciousness in order to capture the chaos that her mind has become and to reconstitute the images that have impinged on it throughout the novel. Mind merges with lurid city to produce a "delirious neon nightscape" (p. 570) through which Flora is pushed and pulled.

What seems to emerge from this psychological mosaic is that Mrs. Hunter has decidedly touched her nurse—not so much with love as with the desire for love, which in Manhood's case is tantamount to the desire for life itself. In giving the sapphire ring to bless the marriage, Mrs. Hunter has recognized Flora's true nature: "She understood me better than anybody ever. I only always didn't like what she dug up out of me" (p. 573). Armorless now, Manhood has paid for the knowledge with pain. A branch cuts across her cheek as she runs from the house in the darkness. It becomes her "wound" (p. 573) and a fugal response to the wound she had inflicted on Mrs. Hunter when she was last dressed in her jewels (p. 540). Manhood has wounded and been wounded, and so is ready for life. These images are accompanied aesthetically and morally by the menstrual blood marking the end of the misconceived, misguided encounter with Mrs. Hunter's son.

"I'm nothing," she tells the pharmacist, to whom she turns out of the nightscape at the end (p. 573). But the truth seems to be that she only feels herself to be nothing because she has lost a no longer defensible self, and the new self is just beginning to grow. Manhood will marry. She will have children—"if the blessed sapphire works" (p. 573). But she will not go back to nursing, having taken from that laboratory profession what she needs: sufficient authenticity to attempt a life of ordinary human love.

Third Shift: Sister de Santis and Transcendence

It is entirely understandable that at the hour of Mrs. Hunter's death, Nurse Manhood should long for the arrival of Mary de Santis, she of the holy name. Whenever the night nurse appears, the novel's life is in the hands of a sanctified woman.

Clothed austerely in her deep blue dress and hat, de Santis suggests authority to her colleagues. She is not quite of them. Literally, that is true because she was born in Athens of a Greek mother and an Italian father. She also has a simple seniority, in that fifteen years before she had been Mrs. Hunter's private nurse during a minor mental breakdown, has nursed her intermittently since then, and now has come "to officiate at the great showdown" (p. 18).

De Santis loves night work. The broad daylight disguises her true nature. With her large breasts and strong calves, White writes, de Santis looks in the daytime as if she were going to play basketball. Nor is she sufficiently articulate to handle the social contacts required in a day nurse. She has the passion but not the speech. At night, however, she unfolds like an angel. Then she can inhabit the shadow and quiet that offer her the sources of wisdom. What is material in the day becomes mysterious in the night when its latent numina shine forth.

At one point de Santis muses about preferring night work because she likes to think highly of people, and, when sleeping, faces "surrender their vices to innocence" (p. 154). That may sound like the sort of remarks parents make in passing, but for de Santis it is working knowledge. She has worked out ways of treating the most vicious patient as if he or she were part of a greater innocence that is found at the end of experience.

The clue to her method is given early. She appears on the opening page of the novel as a nurse who "worked with an air which was not quite professional detachment, nor yet human tenderness; she was probably something of a ritualist" (p. 9). "Not quite professional detachment." That is, she is cool, but not unthinking. That would be Badgery's approach. For de Santis the taking of a temperature has significant meaning apart from the provision of technical data or the requirements of duty. But she has not gone so far as "human tenderness" in the other direction. It is Manhood who is fighting out her life's meaning on that ground. Through ritual—something of a middle way with respect to involvement—de Santis has in a sense gone beyond the human and yet directly into the heart of it.

Once nursing becomes a ritualistic profession, the title "Sister" comes into its own, of course. White makes at least a dozen references to Sister de Santis as a nun. She sees herself as a "votary" (p. 159) always in the novitiate phase (pp. 159, 207, 607); others also see in her dark dress, quiet devotion, and self-effacing manner the demeanor of a nun. Badgery, typically, gets it slightly wrong when she thinks that de Santis has the "smooth, washed look of some of the more simple-minded nuns" (p. 601). Mrs. Hunter's son thinks—again typically, in egotistic, sexual terms—that he has "defiled this pale nun" (p. 356). Mrs. Hunter is closer to the somewhat frightening truth when she identifies both herself and de Santis with conventional attitudes: "Part of you will never be touched. . . . That's what nuns understand, isn't it, Sister?" (p. 445).

But Sister de Santis is not presented as a nursing nun so much as a member of a contemplative order, particularly one that tends a shrine twenty-four hours a day. It is the contemplative whom White has in mind when Mrs. Hunter's son notices that around his mother's prostrate form de Santis moves like an "attendant nun" (p. 152). The patient is de Santis's shrine! And not only hers, but the others' too—the other nurses and the two servants: "The other members of the order, Sisters de Santis and Badgery, and the lay sisters, Lippmann and Cush, were aware it was Sister Manhood who renewed whatever was required for the ritual of anointment" (p. 120).

Manhood may partake of the ritual at times, as she does here during the sacrament of make-up. She may, like de Santis, become a "white-robed priestess" (p. 119) working out "rites" (p. 118). Even Sister Badgery stands at the edge of the order's ritual when she is said to join Mrs. Hunter in a "celebration" at the strength of her pulse (p. 46). But Manhood, as we have seen, opts for human love, and "whatever else, she wouldn't like to be a nun" (p. 115). During the second shift, she toys with specific sacraments as when, for instance, she looks into the toilet bowl "in an attitude of penitence" for evidence of her menstrual blood (p. 539); or when she feels "shriven" at that blood's eventual appearance (p. 551). But her duty is "non-devotional" as compared to de Santis's (p. 538), and de Santis knows why: Manhood has "youth's dread of the sacrosanct" (p. 155). For that reason, though she longs for contact with something beyond herself, "Flora Manhood had never taken part in a mystery: almost . . . if she had been equal to it (less clumsy, ignorant, frightened) with Elizabeth Hunter at moments when the old woman had been willing to share her experience of life" (p. 542).

Manhood remembers once standing at the back of a Catholic church and being intrigued that the bell rung at the transubstantiation signaled that "nothing can become something" (p. 549). Patrick White seems attracted to Catholicism in a similar way. He is intrigued by certain aspects; he will adopt some of the symbols; but his holy nurse, Sister de Santis, is not a Catholic. She had watched her Catholic father become an atheist and be praised for his courage by her Orthodox, icon-dependent—but essentially humanist—mother. Their religion, de Santis realized, had been their deep love for each other. As the only child of this kind of marriage, she had been excluded from the faith and so has had to build one of her own. Her religion has thus grown out of her witnessing of human love—and into an apprehension of the transcendent. That is what de Santis contributes to this novel: a demonstration of how nursing leads to *transcendence*. Whereas in the Catholic mass, the believers are celebrating the creation and resurrection of a body, de Santis's religion enables her to celebrate with Mrs. Hunter the destruction of one. All attest to the fact that "nothing can become something."

This will need to be explained carefully. In the first place, no matter how exalted, de Santis is as human as the other two nurses. When Mrs. Hunter's famous son enters the house, Sister de Santis falls from grace. During the depths of one long night duty, her desire for him causes her to sit in a darkened room and uncover her substantial breasts to the air: an act that is nowhere near the bouncing promiscuity of Sister Manhood, but that nonetheless represents a significant betrayal of de Santis's profession. For virtue, in her case, is linked to an image of nursing as a profession of selflessness. Appropriately, when she first notices her attraction to the son, de Santis's response is to bustle around her patient's room, inventing little jobs "to prove to herself she had not lapsed from the faith" (p. 155). Yet it is in some senses as a nurse that she wishes to offer herself to Mrs. Hunter's son. Nursing and loving are merged for her because she had been nurse to her esteemed father, of whom the son reminds her. She sees them as distinguished but weak men who need love and understanding. Ordinary human love, however, is not meant for her; she transgresses in seeking it. Yet the experience with the son has its spiritual uses in that it keeps her humble, always the novice: "we, the arrogant perfectionists, or pseudo-saints, shall be saved up out of our shortcomings for further trial" (p. 211).

If the possibility of failure is one important element of Sister de Santis's religion, another is the daily reality of suffering, also learned—like the link between nursing and loving—at her father's sickbed. There is a danger of masochism here, of defining selflessness, inaccurately, as the capacity to open one's being wide to another's pain. But the trinity of nursing-love-suffering also holds the possibility of refining clinical empathy to the point of a slender arch rising high above the human fray. Sister de Santis seems to realize all this. There is, at least, a passing reference to the last years of her father's life, during which she, "no longer his daughter or his nurse, had been united with him in a dangerously rarefied climate where love and suffering mingle" (p. 342).

A few years later, de Santis had come to nurse Mrs. Hunter for the first time. At age seventy, her patient still retained the great beauty that had dazzled everyone and seduced many. De Santis, then thirty-five, was not immune, so an acute awareness of physical beauty—and later its startling loss—was added to her religion. The seduction was gentle. "Although you are my nurse . . . I don't want you to emphasize the fact. No ghastly uniform. I'd like people to accept you as my companion. I shall think of you as my friend" (p. 160). This flattering offer from an awesomely beautiful woman turns de Santis not toward human tenderness, but toward ritual: "Mary de Santis had never felt so desperately the need to worship" (p. 167). At first the worship partakes of the aesthetic only. When, for instance, de Santis takes her patient out of the bath and wraps her lovely body in towels, it is her "professional detachment" that saves herself from being "drugged by a pervasive sensuousness," as Manhood might have been. Instead Mrs. Hunter's beauty becomes "an abstraction, in its way far more desirable to anyone hungry for a work of art or of the spirit" (p. 166). If de Santis can turn the beautiful body she is handling into an abstraction, she is well on her way toward her final religious posture. As a mature nurse, she treats all bodies simultaneously on the physical and metaphorical levels as "relics"—sacred objects that remind her of the life within, or, in the sense of "remains," which remind her of the life newly let free. She does not worship the relic—she *tends* the relic—but the life for which it stands.

This mode enables Sister de Santis to regard the loss of Mrs. Hunter's beauty as liberating. The body of the present Mrs. Hunter is simply an "entrance gate" through which both patient and nurse pass to be "exquisitely united . . .[in] a world of trust" (p. 11). They ultimately reach a disembodied state, but the entrance gate must be well tended. It stands as a revelation of the great mystery. The body is a sacramental, if you will, representing the great communion, as in the description of Mrs. Hunter's body as "this precious wafer of flesh" (p. 335). The long passage from which that phrase is taken is worth quoting in its entirety for its remarkable picture of, on the one hand, the superficial sacramentals of the nursing profession, and, on the other, the deeper matter of the spirit that— this is important and not necessarily clear in this particular passage—a ritualistic tending to the superficial will liberate:

> Rational beings are pacified by evidence of efficiency: a scoured bedpan veiled in starched white, the geometry of linen, a temperature chart; or uplifted, rational though they claim to be, by a mystique inherent in the pretty confetti of capsules, and less demonstrative, more insidious, ampoules, locked for safety in the steel cabinet behind the bathroom door. All

of which has only indirect bearing on your significant life, revealed nightly in the presence of this precious wafer of flesh from which earthly beauty has withdrawn, but whose spirit will rise from the bed and stand at the open window, rustling with the light of its own reflections, till finally disintegrating into the white strands strung between the araucarias and oaks of the emergent park, yourself kneeling in spirit to kiss the pearl-embroidered hem, its cold weave the heavier for dew or tears. (p. 335)

Nor is a beautiful mind necessary for worship of the life represented by the patient. It too is only an entrance gate to a transcendental state beyond body and mind. The nurse uses a phrase uttered by a patient, just as she uses the holding of a hand or the wiping of an anus, to achieve entrance into the state. In this ritual the phrase is of no real importance itself because the nurse is reaching for a higher communion. This tenet becomes highly pertinent when the patient is in an unsophisticated neurological state, as is Mrs. Hunter following her stroke. Moreover, what is left of a whole mind can be a "relic" too. But it must not be thought that de Santis is in some way overlooking Mrs. Hunter's present neurological condition. The fact is, neither she nor Mrs. Hunter herself sees it as negative. It is simply another phase of the self, which is constantly in a state of becoming, even in old, old age. That, in one summary, is de Santis's religion— "perpetual becoming" (p. 11). Also, pieces of the mind are lovely in themselves, can be added up, and participate, in some transcendent manner, in the breaking up that reestablishes every kind of life and meaning, as in this attempt by Mrs. Hunter to image that knowledge: "Only yourself and de Santis are real. Only de Santis realizes that the splinters of a mind make a whole piece. Sometimes at night your thoughts glitter; even de Santis can't see that, only yourself: not see, but know yourself to be a detail of the greater splintering" (p. 93).

At this stage personhood does not seem to count for much. The patient and her nurse have moved beyond the body and mind that normally add up to the person. Indeed, they have nearly gone beyond personal existence itself. Now death will mean very little in physical terms. De Santis will not be "emotionally involved by this stage with Mrs Hunter's death" (p. 169). That is due partly to her nursing training: "most of her life she had been personally, though objectively, involved with the physical aspects of death" (p. 353). But mainly her attitude is a religious matter. Looking at her patient's thinning body and thinking of her soul expanding in readiness to leave, de Santis finds Mrs. Hunter "as redemptive as water, as clear as morning light" (p. 12).

In that image the night ends in death just as the morning rises. The image is connected—by the sort of gossamer thread strung throughout this novel—to an incident in which Sister de Santis is walking in the garden among the roses. Her night duty is nearing its end just as she sees a dark, foreign-looking man out for his morning walk. He speaks to her in Greek, her native language, but now almost beyond her ability to translate until finally the meaning comes: "What a sunrise we are making!" (p. 211).

Like the other aspects of her religion, the need to witness to death and its value stems from her experience with her parents, particularly her father. But if religion derives from human need in White's world, it nonetheless carries all the truth de Santis requires. When her father was dying and begging for drugs to relieve the pain, Sister de Santis had given them, against the ethics of her profession ("Love is above ethics": Mrs. Hunter). Her struggle with the ensuing guilt has left her free to see in people's imperfections invitations to deeper connectedness; free to ease the physical pain of dying and the slim line between death and life; and, because of death, free to adore life and its relics. She has her faith:

> On the surface it was her vocation as a nurse. During his worst mental torments Dr Enrico de Santis would ask to see her certificate. He seemed to find comfort in knowing that she was continuing in a tradition. In the final stages he would beg her for the needle, said she had the 'kind touch'. She had obeyed his wishes to the extent of breaking her vows. While Mamma prayed. . . .
> After several years of trial and attempted expurgation, all three had been involved in the great mystery. Mary de Santis, the only survivor, emerged as the votary of life: there were the many others she must save for it; or ease out as she had eased the failed man her father, and her equally failed saint of a mother. (p. 159)

It would seem that de Santis has achieved that quality of wisdom so well defined by Erik H. Erikson as "a detached and yet active concern with life in the face of death."[2] Erikson thinks of wisdom as a potential virtue in old age when death is imminent. But Sister de Santis has looked in the face of death all her professional career. It is nursing that enables her to be *actively* concerned with life in the midst of death; it is her religion, aligned to nursing through ritualizing professional detachment, that enables her to have *detached concern*. De Santis defines love in a way that promotes this detachment: "love is a kind of supernatural state to which I must give myself entirely, and be used up, particularly my imperfections—till I am nothing" (p. 162). In that pure, and utterly passive, receptive state, however—as in the view of Catholicism expressed earlier—nothing can become something very powerful. In this light, even young Manhood's "I'm nothing" (see p. 162 of this essay) suggests spiritual potential.

Living as she does, from time to time de Santis experiences moments of ecstasy. "Unmanageable joy" is what she calls her feeling as she is going through Mrs. Hunter's house for the last time and stops to look into that remarkable old woman's mirror (p. 608). Even after the death of her co-celebrant, de Santis's "veins, her heart, were throbbing with life as she went from room to room throwing open the windows" (p. 607). She thinks of her next patient, an embittered, paraplegic teenager, and wonders "how she would convey to this entombed girl . . . the beauty she herself had witnessed, and love as she had come to understand it" (p. 607). It will not be easy. There will be pain. In fact, the patient has already wounded her—the third such wound in this novel—by willfully sticking a pin into de Santis's outstretched hand. Nurse de Santis may just save her.

Round the Clock

At the core of this vast novel lies the patient. Her stroke notwithstanding, Mrs. Hunter dominates her world. Wealthy, beautiful, and manipulative in her prime, she exudes a peculiar power in her last days. Call it *will* of the most practiced sort. It would not be too much to say that from her horizontal position she commands those who are still vertical. There are several references to her control of the three nurses, even to the point of possessing them in order to get their love. In many ways, Mrs. Hunter is a petty, nasty woman. Yet—and here is the central irony and hope in the novel—it is she who has experienced the eye of the storm on which the title focuses. It is she who has been whirled through life's rubble into the completely serene and deeply connected . . . *nothing* at its center.

This is what de Santis knows about Mrs. Hunter, and what Manhood glimpses. This is what de Santis shares with her, and to some extent learns from her. "Oh nurses!" says Mrs. Hunter. "No end of them. And I'm the one who has to nurse the nurses" (p. 126). The patient—as is sometimes the case—has become the healer.

In the end, she heals the nurses by uniting them. This is accomplished indirectly, after the method of the modern novel. It is nearly axiomatic in modern fiction that the self is many selves and may validly be shown as spread among several characters. And so it is in this novel, in which aspects of Mrs. Hunter are divided among her three nurses.

In her prime Mrs. Hunter had been a social person—not garrulous like Badgery, to be sure, but thoroughly capable of saying the superficial thing to her dinner partner in order to keep the social fabric knitted. Both women are widows as well. Even while her husband lived, in fact, Mrs. Hunter had moved away from him. Like Badgery, Mrs. Hunter can be practical, ostentatiously industrious, and almost "professionally" detached from those around her. And she would have got through life fairly easily with that persona—for, again like Badgery, she plunges into inauthenticity through her acting. But she married and had two children, and that set Mrs. Hunter onto the field where human love must be contested. Like Manhood, she is a sensual woman; like her, too, she has had a terrible ambivalence toward connections that would entrap her. She has not been a warm wife or mother, though she claims to have loved her family, and at the end of his life she nursed her husband not only competently but tenderly. The whole time this woman has lived an inner life as an "eternal aspirant" (p. 102), much like de Santis, as has been shown. Her daughter wonders how "anything of a transcendental nature [could] have illuminated a mind so sensual, mendacious, materialistic, superficial as Elizabeth Hunter's" (p. 589). But it has. She has lived the eye of the storm. She has even become the eye of the storm, and in that manifestation has mingled her spirit with Sister de Santis's. They alone are real at those moments.

Still, the transcendent self is connected to the self that is working out questions of authenticity and to the self concerned with human love. De Santis is connected to Badgery who is connected to Manhood who is connected to de Santis. Shift succeeds shift. Round and round the clock they go: Badgery, Manhood, de Santis, authenticity, human love, transcendence. One must know oneself before one can love others. Through loving others, one may come to apprehend ultimate meaning. Even then, one may find that at the very next moment one is putting on the mask again. It is in the nature of a circle that one can enter it at any point and be, at least potentially, at every point along the circumference.

So it is that the nurses, while they are wearing their uniforms and adopting their professional demeanors, while they are taking the vital signs and emptying the commode, are nonetheless on the path that could take them—through the presence of the patient—to a laboratory where they may learn the nature of human tenderness and on to that place—beyond body, mind, and death itself—at which the clinical virtue of empathy takes on spiritual and joyful significance.

It is a great dance, this circle, a dance around the patient. At one point in the novel, Mrs. Hunter's housekeeper, a former nightclub entertainer now grown old and tarnished, comes into the patient's room to dance a jerky, clenched step for her beloved employer. Round and round she goes. In her hazy state, Mrs. Hunter imagines later that she sees everyone moving around her room: "So they were all dancing: the nurses lined out even skinny Badgery . . ." (p. 446). It is a perfect image for what White's nurses do. The three women, moving through their shifts and their dance, whir into images of mythological types: Badgery into the Woman Who Gives You Birth, Manhood into the One Who Makes Love to You, de Santis into the One Who Buries You. The nurses join hands. Someone is always on duty.

Notes

1. Patrick White, *The Eye of the Storm* (New York: Viking, 1974). All page references are to this edition and will be cited parenthetically in the text.
2. Erik H. Erikson, "Life Cycle," *International Encyclopedia of the Social Sciences* 9 (1968): 292.

Part III

Issues and Images

The essays in Part III all deal in various ways with the complex interactions between images of nurses and the broader social issues of twentieth-century America: racism, sexism, and the reductionism of popular culture. The ordering of these essays reflects the historical development of our social concern. In American culture, the pernicious effects of racism were recognized and addressed in the civil rights movement of the 1960s. It was almost a decade later before the similar pernicious effects of sexism were recognized and addressed by the women's rights movement. The raised social consciousness that resulted from these two movements caused scholars to begin to study how popular images in the mass media reflect and shape general social attitudes toward racial minorities and women. The first essay in Part III, then, focuses on the intersection of images of nurses and images of blacks. The second essay examines the interaction between images of nurses and the general social conditioning and stereotyping of women. The third and final essay looks at an example of the way general attitudes toward women in a particular era influence the creation of a popular image, even when the image is based on historical fact.

In the first essay of Part III, "'They Shall Mount Up with Wings as Eagles': Historical Images of Black Nurses, 1890–1950," Darlene Clark Hine describes the historical dilemma of black nurses, who had to contend with two conflicting images: respected and admired within the black community, they endured overt racial discrimination by the white community, including white nurses, who maintained an image of black nurses as professional inferiors. Hine examines how these racially motivated negative images influenced the personal and professional development of the black nurse, using as her examples the lives of Mary Elizabeth Lancaster Carnegie, Frances Elliott Davis, Mabel Keaton Staupers, and Eunice Rivers (Laurie). Hine also discusses the role of the National Association of Colored Graduate Nurses and the more recent National Black Nurses' Association in helping black nurses overcome the racial injustices perpetuated even within the world of professional nursing itself by negative images of blacks.

In the second essay, "Of Images and Ideals: A Look at Socialization and Sexism in Nursing," Janet Muff discusses the integral relationship between the historical problems of nursing and the issues of women in a traditionally male-dominated society. She argues, perhaps controversially, that nurses themselves are responsible for the current difficulties of their profession and that nurses can solve their problems, but only if they begin recognizing women's issues as nursing's issues. After an extensive discussion of the impact external social and political forces—socialization, sexism, and stereotyping—have had on nurses and nursing, Muff examines the stress of nurses and the conflicts within the profession that result from the disjunction between the ideal and the reality of nursing. Muff ends her essay with recommendations for action nurses can take to combat the effects of sexism and improve their profession and the way it is perceived.

"*The White Angel* (1936): Hollywood's Image of Florence Nightingale," by Anne Hudson Jones, closes Part III and the book with an examination of the popular image of Florence Nightingale as presented in this film, which was formally endorsed by the American Nurses' Association. Based on Lytton Strachey's biography of Nightingale, the film alters facts and modifies Nightingale's image to fit the pattern of the working-girl movies of the 1930s; yet the essential archetypal images of nurses persist, and Nightingale is identified iconographically as mother, seductress, and saintly secular nun. In creating a popular and palatable image for mass consumption, the filmmakers simplified Nightingale's character, thus idealizing her and diminishing her at the same time. This reduction of Nightingale from powerful woman to popular heroine is only one example of the continuous transformation of women as old images and the social needs of a particular era (for women to stay at home, or go to work, or go to war, or whatever) intersect. More subtle than propaganda, well-made popular films such as *The White Angel* exert an important influence on their viewers. When such films are promoted and widely promulgated as "educational," their images can become more influential than the historical reality on which they are based.

Darlene Clark Hine

8. "They Shall Mount Up with Wings as Eagles": Historical Images of Black Nurses, 1890–1950

Although diverse and often contradictory images of nurses permeate American society, few writers have investigated or dissected the particular images of black nurses. Two general images of the professional black nurse prevailed during the first half of twentieth-century America. The black nurse was viewed, on the one hand, as an essential and competent provider of health care in black communities. She, more than most other health care personnel, was viewed as being completely responsive to the needs of black people. Within the largely segregated communities, the black nurse represented an uncompromising voice speaking out for the best interests of blacks. On the other hand, the black nurse was perceived as an inferior member of the nursing profession when compared to her white counterparts. The image of the black nurse as an inferior professional was created and reinforced by discriminatory treatment. Accordingly, she was subjected to employment discrimination, educational segregation, economic exploitation, professional exclusion, and social abuse. The real-life experiences of four black nurses, Mary Elizabeth Lancaster Carnegie, Frances Elliott Davis, Mabel Keaton Staupers, and Eunice Rivers (Laurie), enhance our understanding of the dual processes of image formation and transformation.

On an eventful day in 1942, Mary Elizabeth Lancaster Carnegie, a black nurse, reported for duty as a clinical instructor at the St. Philip Hospital, the separate Negro wing of the white-controlled Medical College of Virginia. Carnegie had earned her diploma in 1937 from the segregated Lincoln School of Nurses in New York City. After graduation, she worked for several years as a general-duty nurse at the black Veterans Administration Hospital in Tuskegee, Alabama, before receiving a Bachelor of Arts degree in 1942 from the West Virginia State College. In spite of her previous nursing experience and unique academic preparation, Carnegie, recalling that unforgettable day at St. Philip, wrote: "Here began my first in-training lessons in what it means to be a Negro nurse in the South."[1]

In keeping with long-established patterns of racial etiquette, all the white administrators, physicians, and nurses at St. Philip addressed white nurses as "Miss" and black nurses as "Nurse." This practice underscored the inferior status of black nurses and the low esteem in which they were held by white co-workers. Yet, as Carnegie noted, being called "Nurse so-and-so" was "a step up from being addressed by first names. . . ."[2] As if to compound their subordination, however, Carnegie observed: "Not only were Negro nurses addressed this way by the white nurses and doctors, they were instructed to address each other and refer to themselves in this manner."[3] Refusing to acquiesce to this social affront and professional slight, Carnegie declared to her black co-workers, "You can't control what someone else does, but you can control what you do."[4] Unmindful of the consequences and perhaps suspecting that her tenure at St. Philip would be brief, Carnegie admonished the black student nurses to "address themselves and each other as 'Miss.'"[5] She insisted that the black students extend this courtesy and manifest respect by addressing all their black patients as "Miss, Mrs., or Mr.," in spite of the fact that white nurses and doctors also addressed the Negro patients by their first names.

Carnegie's head-on collision with symbolic racism as reflected in the denial of appropriate titles to black women nurses was one small skirmish in a decades-long war for professional recognition and acceptance. Between 1893, when the first group of professionaly trained black nurses appeared, and 1951, the year of the dissolution of the National Association of Colored Graduate Nurses (NACGN), founded in 1908, black nurse leaders had struggled on every conceivable front to win equal pay, access to better quality training institutions, admission into advanced educational programs, broader employment opportunities, and individual membership in the American Nurses' Association. Progress toward these objectives and the eradication of the image of professional inferior was slow, as deeply entrenched negative white perceptions, attitudes, and actions toward black nurses halted advance.[6]

Actually, the many discriminatory practices of key American institutions, such as the United States military establishment and organized nursing bodies, contributed to the growth of negative images of black nurses and reinforced the already low esteem in which many whites held them.

The American Red Cross's treatment of Frances Elliott Davis, a 1912 graduate of the black Freedmen's Hospital training school in Washington, D.C., is but one illustration of this point. Davis was the first black nurse to secure enrollment in the American Red Cross. At the end of World War I all nurses, with one exception, received identical pins indicating their enrollment and service in the Red Cross. However, the pin given to Davis was marked "1A," indicating that she was the first black nurse to be enrolled in the Red Cross. Thereafter, beginning with Frances Elliott Davis, from 1918 to 1949, all Negro nurses enrolled in the American Red Cross received special pins with the letter "A" inscribed.[7]

To be sure, Davis could have refused to accept the Red Cross pin with its discriminatory inscription. She had protested against segregation and other humiliating practices throughout her career. On her first Red Cross assignment in Jackson, Tennessee, Davis had pointedly objected to her white supervisor's introducing her to patients and co-workers as "Fannie." Moreover, she had successfully challenged the local custom requiring black patients and black health care personnel to enter the local hospital through the back door. Yet, when presented with the choice of accepting or rejecting the differently marked pin, Davis acquiesced. She swallowed her pride, accepted the pin, and consoled herself with the knowledge that she had, at least, opened a previously closed door through which other black nurses would enter. In short, to advance the professional interests of black nurses she chose to put aside personal considerations. As her biographer maintains, Davis ultimately could not "turn her back . . . simply because she had to face a certain amount of humiliation from white people who thought themselves superior."[8]

While Davis endured silently, the advent of World War II created a fortuitous array of circumstances that enabled some black nurses under the leadership of Mabel Keaton Staupers to protest loudly historical patterns of institutional racism and discrimination. Staupers, a 1917 graduate of the Freedmen's Hospital School of Nursing and executive secretary of the NACGN, took advantage of the war emergency and the increased demand for nurses to improve the status and image of black nurses as competent and valuable health care givers. Early on, War Department officials had declared that black nurses would not be called to serve in the Armed Forces Nurse Corps. As a result of pressures and protests from organized nursing groups skillfully orchestrated by Staupers, the army soon modified this policy and, in January 1941, announced that a quota of fifty-six black nurses would be recruited and assigned to the black military installations at Camp Livingston in Louisiana and Fort Bragg in North Carolina. Navy officials remained intransigent, and the Navy Nurse Corps continued to exclude black nurses throughout the war years.[9]

Staupers readily conceded that the army's quota of fifty-six represented an advance over World War I practices of total exclusion. Yet she remained determined to continue the assault on all such barriers. From 1941 to 1945 Staupers met repeatedly with white nursing groups, top military officials, first lady Eleanor Roosevelt, and leaders of black civil rights organizations. She cultivated relations with editors of black newspapers, women's clubs, and white philanthropists, urging them to protest the imposition of quotas for black nurses.[10] Her strategic maneuvering eventually bore fruit.

The personal appeals of Eleanor Roosevelt and the protests of the National Nursing Council for War Service, combined with the acute nurse shortage toward the end of the war, eventually forced the army to increase the numbers of black nurses. By 1945, approximately 330 black nurses were serving in the Army Nurse Corps. Had black nurses been accepted in proportion to their numbers, as were white nurses, there would have been 1,520 of them in the Army and Navy Nurse Corps. There were at the time approximately eight thousand black graduate nurses active in nursing.[11] Unable to withstand the unrelenting pressure, the surgeon general of the navy declared on January 31, 1945: "There is no policy in the Navy which discriminates against the utilization of Negro Nurses."[12]

Although the American Red Cross, the United States Army and Navy, and some white nurses and doctors discriminated against black nurses, viewing them as inferior professionals, the black community's general reactions to and perceptions of black nurses were strikingly different. In part, this divergence is explained by the insufficient health care available to large portions of the black population. The small numbers of black physicians, coupled with a growing trend to concentrate in urban areas, and the frequently insulting treatment meted out by white physicians often meant that only a black nurse was available in most rural communities.[13] In many such areas, rural black nurses, similar to Eunice Rivers (Laurie), a 1922 graduate of Tuskegee Institute's nursing program in Tuskegee, Alabama, played a pivotal role in the black health care delivery hierarchy in rural Alabama.

Rivers attributed the higher esteem that the black nurses found among blacks to the position they occupied as mediators between patients and physicians. Historian James H. Jones, in his provocative study of the Tuskegee syphilis experiment conducted by the United States Public Health

Service (1932–1972), underscored the significant role played by Nurse Rivers. Her immense interpersonal skills won the trust and respect of hundreds of the male patients involved in the experiment. Jones describes Rivers as "a facilitator, bridging the many barriers that stemmed from the educational and cultural gap between the physicians and the subjects."[14] In one interview, Rivers elaborated on her image of the role the black nurse played:

> . . . the doctor saw the patient and he was gone and it was up to you to help that patient carry out his orders, do whatever the doctor suggested. The doctor said you do so and so. . . . First thing, the patient doesn't know how to do it. He doesn't know what his reaction is going to be. He doesn't want to be stuck. . . . So the nurse plays an important part there. She's closer to the patient. Patients would get to the point where if they're not sure, they're going to ask you. They get you in the middle.[15]

Rivers recalled, "A lot of my patients would not call a doctor until I had come to see them, to see how they were doing and see if they needed a doctor." She added, "I had an awful time training them to go ahead and get their own doctor."[16]

These capsule glimpses into the experiences of Carnegie, Davis, Staupers, and Rivers provoke more questions than answers concerning both the images of black women and the reality of their struggles as professional nurses. Why were black nurses denied the usual appellations denoting respect? Why were they given Red Cross pins inscribed with the letter "A"? Why did the United States Army and Navy first exclude black nurses altogether, as in World War I, and then, in World War II, establish quotas for recruiting them into the Armed Forces Nurse Corps? In light of the demeaning treatment accorded them in the larger society, why were black nurses held in such high esteem within the black community? What did the black community expect and receive from black nurses? Finally, how did discrimination, racism, and negative stereotypes spur or impede the personal and professional development of the black nurse?

Traditional histories of nursing pay scant attention to the accomplishments and peculiar difficulties encountered by black nurses. Yet the struggle of black nurses for respect, recognition, acceptance, and status parallels and, in many ways, exemplifies the historical quest of all professional nurses. It is the difference that race made, giving rise to a store of derogatory images, which separates and distinguishes the black nurses' story from the larger history. Examining some of the historical images of black nurses and contrasting them with the objective reality provide deeper insights into the process of professionalization in nursing. Such an investigation enhances our understanding of the old images that American pioneer nursing leaders desired to destroy and the new ones that they substituted. In the years of the early professionalization, concerned nursing leaders initiated actions designed to limit the number of nurses, halt the proliferation of training schools, and recruit "women of the better classes" into the profession. From the outset, the quest for image control and exclusiveness in nursing were essential components and characteristics of the overall professionalization process.[17]

Unfortunately, black women, and lower-class white women to some extent, were most affected by exclusionary tendencies and hence were sacrificed on the altar of nursing advancement. As nursing increasingly acquired the trappings of a profession, the restrictions and impediments placed in the paths of black women mushroomed. They were denied admittance into training schools, barred from membership in professional associations, refused listing in employment registries, and discouraged from aspiring to meet the higher requirements of nurse registration and licensing laws. Black women, because of their racial identity and slavery heritage, were seen as a permanently alien and inferior group that could not be assimilated. In the white mind the slavery-born images of the black woman as a defeminized beast of burden, a sexually promiscuous wanton, or a domineering mammy held sway long after the demise of the "peculiar institution." These negative images, mixed with entrenched racism, probably motivated those of the white nursing establishment seeking greater status and esteem to eschew association with or recognition of black women as professional peers.[18] Before I proceed, it will be useful to place these images of black women and nurses within the appropriate historical context.

In the latter part of the nineteenth century, the social conventions and normative attitudes of an industrialized society consigned women to the private sphere of the home. The ideology of "virtuous womanhood" sharply and oppressively defined their proper actions and behavior in very narrow and restricted terms. Women were considered to be repositories of moral sensibility, purity, refinement, and maternal affection in a male-dominated society. Thus, woman's highest calling consistent with her biological destiny was deigned to be that of mother and nurturer. For many women, growing adherence to the ideology of separate spheres occurred in tandem with constricting career opportunities in the public sphere of business and politics. Actually, the tension between theory and reality created a paradox, for as certain doors closed, other new female-stereotyped occupations and professions reserved for women opened.[19]

Of all such sex-segregated occupations, nursing was preeminent. The movement for formalized nursing training and practice provided an attractive alternative to middle-class, sphere-restricted women. Before the Civil War, nursing, as historian Janet Wilson James has pointed out, was a "low-paid, low-status job for laboring class women, who, over a twelve-hour day, attended to the physical needs of the patients while doing the heavy domestic work on the wards."[20] The opening of the first nursing schools, in 1873, launched the movement to upgrade nursing, to distance it from identification with domestic service, and to attract a "higher-class woman" into the profession. Traditionally considered a woman's job, nursing neither threatened nor challenged society's views of her traditional domestic functions. Rather, the substance of nursing and settings in which training was provided actually reinforced the image of the subordinate woman. Deemed less exacting and autonomous than medicine, nursing existed always under the control of the male-dominated medical and hospital professions.[21]

The late nineteenth- and early twentieth-century struggle to professionalize and upgrade the image of nursing concentrated, in part, on recruiting middle-class students while purging and excluding from the occupation the uneducated and untrained women of the lower socioeconomic classes. These efforts also coincided with the hardening of the color line in American society. As segregation pervaded the country, all southern and most northern nursing schools barred black women. Even in the most liberal northern institutions black women were subjected to restrictive quotas. The charter for the New England Hospital for Women and Children, for example, expressly stipulated that only *one* Negro and *one* Jewish student each year would be accepted. The first black trained nurse, Mary E. Mahoney, was graduated from the New England Hospital in 1879.[22]

If black women were to have access to professional nursing training, then it was incumbent on black leaders, in the name of racial self-help, to establish the corresponding institutions. Beginning in the early 1890s, black physician Daniel Hale Williams of Chicago and educator Booker T. Washington, founder of Tuskegee Institute, spearheaded a movement to found hospital nursing schools for black women. They solicited operating funds for these new institutions from their respective black communities and from private philanthropies. The rhetoric of the founders of the early black nursing schools reveals much about their own and the larger society's images of nurses. Washington and Williams espoused the new romantic and idealized image of the Florence Nightingale-type nurse. They merged this image with their views of what constituted the "proper" woman's role. Uppermost in their minds, however, was the belief that the black woman bore a large part of the responsibility for proving the humanity of black people to a skeptical white public. Accordingly, they portrayed the black nurse as a self-sacrificing, warm, and devoted mother figure, and downplayed her as the efficient, autonomous, and assertive professional. Fund-raising campaigns for the hospitals and training schools employing this romantic image of the black nurse-mother proved most successful. Evoking this romantic image had other practical implications as well. Clearly, the black nurses trained in these black community-based and supported institutions would forever owe primary allegiance to blacks and be responsible participants in the climb up the racial and social ladder.[23]

Williams, as founder of two black nursing schools, Provident Hospital and Training School in Chicago in 1891 and the Freedmen's Hospital nursing school in Washington, D.C., in 1894, frequently informed potential black supporters of nursing schools: "The servant class no longer furnishes the nurse."[24] Ironically, Williams was prone to invoke the ubiquitous "mammy" image to illustrate his claim that the black woman was a "natural" nurse possessed of a long heritage, in slavery and freedom, of caring for the sick of both races. He was, perhaps, unmindful that this continued association of black nurses with the mammy image would retard their advancement within the nursing profession. Williams insisted: "The young colored woman who chooses this calling enters the training school richly endowed by inheritance with woman's noblest attributes—fidelity, tenderness, sympathy."[25] After extolling all the nurturing qualities of black women, Williams declared the black nurse an object lesson, who "teaches the people cleanliness, thrift, habits of industry, sanitary housekeeping, the proper care of themselves, and of their children. She teaches them how to prepare food, the selection of proper clothing for the sick and the well, and how to meet emergencies."[26] As Rivers would do thirty years later, Williams predicted that the trained black nurse would soon become a major force serving the black community in racial uplift work.[27]

Booker T. Washington, when launching the nursing program at Tuskegee Institute in 1892, linked it with the school's industrial education emphasis. He justified the new program on the grounds that nursing training would enable a black woman to have a career prior to marriage, one, however, that would also make her a better wife, mother, and home-maker. Moreover, he argued that should hard times befall the family, the trained nurse would always be able to help earn money. In describing the philosophical foundation on which the school was based, Washington re-iterated tenets of the Victorian belief concerning woman's role and func-tion: "A man can build the house but the woman must, for the most part, furnish the sort of culture and refinement that makes it a home," he said.[28] Washington wedded nursing training firmly to vocational work: "The course in child nurture and nursing has been established to complete the training in home building which is carried on as part of the industrial training of young women at Tuskegee."[29]

Williams's and Washington's images of the black nurse were shared for many years by most black hospital administrators and physicians respon-sible for their training. In a 1918 article, John A. Kenney, a black physician named superintendent of the new and enlarged John A. Andrew Memorial Hospital and Nurse Training School of Tuskegee Institute, echoed Wil-liams and Washington's conviction that the black nurse was equal, if not superior, to white nurses. In an effort to persuade more black women to enter into the backbreaking, endless toil euphemistically referred to as nursing training, he unabashedly lauded the black nurses' many womanly virtues of "devotion, endurance, sympathy, tactile delicacy, unselfishness, tact, resourcefulness, [and] willingness to undergo hardships. . . ."[30] The fact that he played an important role in training black women did not challenge Kenney to view the trained nurse as a serious professional rather than a mother-nurturer. Even when commenting on the good deeds per-formed by the black graduate nurses of Tuskegee Institute, Kenney inter-jected remembrances of his mother's unpaid nurturing activities. He wrote: "Regardless of the demands made upon her by the exacting duties of her own household, if there was a case of serious illness among her friends, white or colored, even miles away, she thought it her duty to go and care for them night after night, if necessary."[31]

The black nurse was entrapped in the vortex of the sexual and racial currents dominating black and white thought in late nineteenth-century America. To be sure, at this juncture much of the language describing black nurses and the "advantages" to be reaped by pursuing a nursing career were used with white women as well. Although reality and image frequently diverged, nevertheless, the ideology of separate spheres severely reduced a woman's chances for challenging and remunerative work. Because of racial prejudice, most of the sex-segregated jobs were beyond the black woman's reach. The transformation of nursing into a skilled profession requiring formal training in a structured institutional setting further encumbered the black woman. With black women barred from the white nursing schools, black leaders, in order to provide access to the profession, proceeded to combine the ideology of woman's separate sphere with the doctrine of racial uplift. Thus, because the black communities contributed so much to the start-up funds creating and sustaining the black nursing schools, the early generations of graduates were expected to repay the communities' investments. Hence, in addition to seeking professional acceptance and recognition, the black nurse bore the extra burden of providing health care for, and lifting up from the bottom of the American social scale, the entire black race. All future images in the black mind of the black woman nurse would be inextricably connected to her role within, and responsibility to, the black community.

By the 1920s, the separate black training schools had produced approximately three thousand nurses. The burgeoning numbers caused white nurses, especially those engaged in private-duty work, to fear increased economic competition, which only exacerbated the tenuous relations between the two groups. Meanwhile, economic exigencies and racism compelled many black nurses to act in ways that reinforced existing negative images of them in the minds of their white colleagues. For example, many black nurses worked for lower wages and longer hours than white nurses. Often, black nurses performed household and child-care chores in addition to tending to sick members of a family. The fact that many white physicians spoke in glowing terms of the submissive and accommodating black nurse who adapted "well to the needs of the household" did not help matters.[32] Equally damaging were their expressions of delight with black private-duty nurses, whom they perceived as being more "willing to render the small personal services only grudgingly performed by white nurses."[33] In a depressed job market, characterized by an oversupply of nurses and decreasing patient demands, black nurses were imagined as being the group least committed to advancing the profession and more willing to compromise on salary and working conditions.[34]

The scarcity of data precludes the development of a definitive analysis of white nurses' images of black nurses during the 1920s. Available, however, are a limited number of surveys and reports commissioned by philanthropic and nursing organizations, which canvassed white nurses, physicians, and hospital and public health officials for their personal evaluations and perceptions of the black nurse. In 1925, Ethel Johns, an Englishwoman trained in a Canadian hospital, conducted one of the most illuminating surveys and reports. Under the aegis of the Rockefeller Foundation, Johns queried hundreds of white administrators and nurse superintendents in more than two dozen hospitals and visited scores of visiting nursing associations and municipal boards of health.

Johns's report, though frozen in time, does record the attitudes of the black nurses' professional colleagues while shedding light on the black nurses' social and economic status. The images white nurses and other health care personnel had of black nurses were informed by the widely held assumption of the poor quality of all black training schools. Moreover, the fact that blacks as a group occupied a subordinate position in America influenced the negative assessments of their leadership abilities. Most of the white superintendents of the twenty-three black hospitals Johns visited frankly admitted their displeasure with black nurses. They contended that black nurses exhibited "a marked tendency to concealment of what is going on in their respective wards. They will not report mistakes or accidents. . . ."[35] These claims, while perhaps accurate, did not take into consideration the forces that may have encouraged black nurses to cover for each other when a white supervisor was overhead. Few black nurses held supervisory positions in hospitals or sanitariums. Without dissecting the underlying reasons for the absence of black nurse administrators, Johns simply concluded that they were inherently lacking in leadership qualities: "My observations lead me to believe that the negro woman is temperamentally unsuited for the constant unremitting grind of a hospital superintendent's life. She finds it difficult to discipline her staff and yet to remain on friendly terms with them."[36]

While black nurse supervisors were scarce, the chances of black nurses for employment in the public health field during the 1920s were even more bleak. Visiting nursing association officials rationalized their aversion to hiring black public health nurses, insisting that they were of limited usefulness. Most agency leaders maintained that black nurses could work only with blacks, but white public health nurses could deal with both races. After all, these officials contended, black nurses were educationally deficient and ill prepared to assume the heavy responsibility of being a public health nurse. Supervisors of the nursing services for the municipal boards of health in New York, Chicago, and Philadelphia acknowledged that, as much as possible, they hired only white nurses because the employment of blacks "complicates the service and creates social friction."[37] Municipal boards of health supervisors in Birmingham, Baltimore, Atlanta, and Nashville regarded the black public health nurse as "admittedly inferior in intelligence to the white group. . . ."[38] They let it be known that, where employed, the black nurse was "paid substantially less than the white nurse. . . . excluded from supervisory rank and . . . treated as a social inferior. . . ."[39]

Several directors of visiting nursing services did comment positively on the role of black nurses in public health nursing. Lillian Wald, founder of the Henry Street Settlement and a staunch friend of black nurses, employed 25 black and 150 white nurses, paid them equal salaries, and accorded them identical professional courtesies and recognition. Even here, however, black and white nurses were viewed and treated differently in two respects: black nurses were never sent to white homes, nor were they promoted to supervisory rank. Johns discovered similar conditions prevailing in Philadelphia, Chicago, and Saint Louis. Southern-based visiting nurse services employed black nurses; nevertheless, when they were hired they always received much lower salaries and were treated as social inferiors.[40]

Among the whites interviewed, Johns discerned nearly unanimous agreement that the black nurse was a professional inferior. According to most white nurses, supervisors, and administrators, the lower wages paid black nurses were entirely justified and simply confirmed alleged black shortcomings. The fact that black nurses were rarely promoted to or held supervisory and administrative positions reinforced white beliefs that blacks were incapable of leading. Only when she dealt with black patients did the black nurse stand a chance of being referred to as a competent and adept professional. Apparently, only as long as she remained in the black community, caring only for black patients, would the black nurse earn praise from her white counterparts and enjoy a better image. Johns well captured these mixed messages when she observed:

> It is quite apparent that the negro nurse cannot be utilized successfully in public health work except among her own people. Even among them she has not the same authority as the white nurse although she has a better psychological approach. She has been very successful in overcoming their superstitious fears regarding immunization, vaccination and other preventive measures. The social and economic problems involved in case work are commonly too much for her but she can ferret out information and interpret

domestic complications which would baffle a white nurse who lacks her intuitive understanding of racial characteristics.[41]

Fortunately, black nurses were highly regarded within black urban and rural communities. For thousands of poor blacks the nurse often meant the difference between living and dying. The black nurse allayed the fears and quelled the hostilities of those superstitious rural blacks who refused to seek medical care in hospitals and usually resorted to folk cures and questionable remedies. Frequently, the black nurse became the bridge connecting rural impoverished blacks mired in nineteenth-century notions of sickness with the twentieth-century reality of hospitals, physicians, scientific advances, and the germ theory of disease.[42]

Actually, the image of the race-serving, strong, and resourceful black nurse laboring amongst the poor and downtrodden is too one-dimensional. Eunice Rivers, to be specific, was described by her family, friends, colleagues, and black patients as a "born nurse." She had entered nursing out of a desire "to get closer to people who needed" her. Rivers attributed her success as a nurse to an innate ability to accept people on their own terms. She stated in an interview, "I go there and visit awhile until I know when to make some suggestions. . . . I don't ever go into any person's house, fussing with him about how he keeps his house, first." Rivers insisted, "I accepted them as they were and they accepted me."[43]

Rivers was more than a good country nurse. Her more than forty years' involvement in the Tuskegee syphilis experiment, in which treatment was deliberately withheld from patients, raises questions concerning relationships between the black nurses and the black community and between black nurses and white health care professionals. Indeed, it is fair to say that without her the white "government doctors" would not have been successful in engaging so many black males in such a detrimental and ethically bankrupt experiment. It was their unquestioning faith in Rivers as someone selflessly looking out for and protecting them that led the men to continue in the experiment for so many unrewarding years. Though they remained fundamentally suspicious of the "government doctors'" motives, they always tended to do what Rivers told them. According to historian James H. Jones, "more than any other person, [Rivers] made them believe that they were receiving medical care that was helping them."[44] They were not.

Nurse Rivers's motives for collaborating in this experiment and deliberately manipulating these black men are complex. It is possible that Rivers viewed the experiment as a way of ensuring for at least some blacks an unparalleled amount of medical attention. Jones offers several compelling explanations for Rivers' complicity: As a nurse, Rivers had been trained to follow orders and probably it simply did not occur to her to question a, or for that matter any, doctor's judgment. Moreover, she was incapable of judging the scientific merits of the study. For Rivers, a female in a male-dominated world, deference to male authority figures reinforced her ethical passivity. Finally, and perhaps most significantly, Rivers was black and the physicians who controlled the experiment were white. Years of conditioning and living in the South made it virtually impossible for Rivers to have rebelled against a white male government doctor, the ultimate authority figure in her world.[45] In this case the needs and interests of the black community of Tuskegee were not addressed and protected by the black nurse.

The image of the black nurse as self-sacrificing mother-nurturer, servant, and leader of the black community persisted with slight modifications. In the urban northern black communities the white uniform-clad black nurse with satchel at her side cut an imposing and impressive figure. One black nurse, Elizabeth Jones, recounted ways in which the black community viewed the black nurse as someone special. She describes, for example, her own approach one day to two children playing on a Harlem street. One child, as she walked toward them, ordered his playmates, "'Get up, and let the lady pass.' While making a passage, all eyes were turned upon [her] with great intent. Suddenly, as if having solved a problem, one little voice chimed in, and said with much glee, 'Aw! She ain't a lady, she's a nurse!'"[46] Jones, musing about this reflection on the status of the black nurse in the black community, declared: "Not only is she a teacher, but she is looked upon by most of those with whom she comes in contact, as an example of the higher life."[47] For many blacks the black nurse became a symbol of white middle-class virtues and respectability. Residents of the black communities where the nurse visited, worked, and sometimes resided looked upon her with pride tinged with awe. The fact that she was there to tend to their needs and to help them solve their problems engendered feelings of possessiveness while intensifying desires to obey.

Throughout the brief history of professional nursing, black nurses struggled to create and sustain positive self-images while simultaneously pursuing an often frustrating quest for acceptance and recognition within their chosen occupation. Accommodation to their "place" and resistance to white efforts to devalue them developed as two forms of a single process by which black nurses accepted circumstances they could not change and vigorously fought individually and collectively for professional equality.

Throughout her long nursing career, Red Cross nurse Davis demonstrated pride and a positive self-image. Her deep spiritual convictions and unyielding sense of responsibility to her race, combined with the support and love of her husband, sustained her quest for professional equality. These internal and external forces helped to deflect the psychological and moral aggression of a racist society. When gloom threatened to immobilize and depress her, she invariably reached for her Bible and reread her favorite passage from the Book of Isaiah: "But they that wait upon the Lord shall renew their strength; they shall mount up with wings as eagles; they shall run, and not be weary; and they shall walk, and not faint" (40:31).[48]

Mabel Keaton Staupers was thirteen years old when her family moved from Barbados, West Indies, in 1903, to the Harlem community of New York City. She spent the early years of her nursing career in New York City and Washington, D.C.; in 1920, in cooperation with a couple of prominent black physicians, she organized the Booker T. Washington Sanatorium, the first facility in the Harlem area where black physicians could treat their patients. In 1921 she was awarded a working fellowship in Philadelphia and was later assigned to the chest department of the Jefferson Hospital Medical College in Philadelphia. The following year Staupers returned to New York, and under the auspices of the New York Tuberculosis and Health Association, she made a survey of the health needs of the community, which eventually resulted in the organization of the Harlem Committee of the New York Tuberculosis and Health Association and her twelve-year stint as executive secretary of this body.[49]

In 1934 Staupers was appointed as the first nurse executive of the National Association of Colored Graduate Nurses (NACGN). Founded in 1908 by a group of black nurses in New York, the organization was virtually moribund by the time Staupers assumed the helm. Throughout the 1940s Staupers combined her struggle for the integration of black nurses into the Armed Forces Nurse Corps with the fight for full integration of black nurses into American nursing. In 1948 the American Nurses' Association (ANA) House of Delegates opened the doors to individual black membership, appointed a black woman nurse as assistant executive secretary in its national headquarters, and witnessed the election of black nurse Estelle Massey Riddle to the Board of Directors. In 1950 the NACGN membership elected Staupers president. The NACGN's Board of Directors charged Staupers with overseeing the dissolution of the organization. Her book, *No Time for Prejudice* (1961), details the history of the black nurses' victorious struggle to integrate into the American Nurses' Association.[50]

The fight for integration into state nurses' associations in the South continued even after the ANA openly accepted black members on an individual basis. Mary Elizabeth Lancaster Carnegie led the attack against the Florida State Nurses Association. After leaving St. Philip, Carnegie worked as assistant director of the Division of Nurse Education at Hampton Institute in Virginia. In 1945 she was named Dean of the Division of Nursing Education at Florida A & M College. In 1951 Carnegie received a fellowship to earn a master's degree from Syracuse University in New York. She was assistant editor of the *American Journal of Nursing* from 1953 to 1956, then became associate editor and, in 1970, editor of *Nursing Outlook*. While pursuing her editorial career, Carnegie was a part-time student at New York University, where she received a doctoral degree in 1972. The next year she assumed the editorship of *Nursing Research*.[51]

Carnegie's somewhat exceptional career was unlike that of most black nurses; yet even her advancement was profoundly impeded by racist attitudes and discrimination. A clearly hostile larger social environment littered her path with innumerable reminders of her status as a Negro nurse. Carnegie, however, deliberately chose to resist those practices that assaulted her self-image. Carnegie's description of the black nurses' struggle for the right to participate in the meetings of the Florida State Nurses Association illuminates the strength of their determination to win professional recognition and acceptance and the ludicrous nature of the efforts of some white nurses to preserve segregation and subordination: "For many months, we played a game of 'musical chairs'. The white nurses would wait on the outside of the buildings for us to arrive and be seated; then they would proceed to sit on the opposite side of the meeting room. If we sat in the back, they would sit in the front, and vice versa."[52] Carnegie devised a clever scheme to end "the game." She and her fellow black nurses simply waited for the white nurses to arrive and would scatter throughout the room in order to ensure, at least, integration in the seating arrangements. When, in 1950, she was elected to the board for a three-year term, she continued to press quietly for integration. After the 1950 meeting Carnegie observed that "for the first time, all Negro nurses attended all business and programme meetings, but were barred from the luncheon."[53] By the 1952 convention in Daytona Beach, Florida, she reported modest improvements: "There was integration in every respect but housing and the events that were strictly social."[54] (The luncheon meetings at the hotel included all members on an equal basis.)

By the 1950s it was evident that the self-image of the black nurse was formed in part by the twin realities of racism and sexism in American society. Black nurses recognized that their struggle for recognition, acceptance, and equality of opportunity within nursing was inextricably linked to overcoming this double-edged prejudice. Carnegie captured the relationship between the development of a positive self-image and struggle for unfettered access to professional opportunities when she asserted: "In the length and breadth of the United States of America, Negro nurses, many unknown to each other, have always fought for a common cause. . . . They were fighting on the same front in schools of nursing and in professional organizations in other states, and on other fronts—in the military, public health, hospital nursing service, industry, private duty, and the national organizations—throughout the country."[55] Actually, the dual processes of accommodation and resistance enabled black nurses to develop a collective self-consciousness and pride that allowed them to retain a viable sense of self-worth in the face of the oppression they endured. Central to their identity, however, was a strong conviction that, in the words of black nurse educator-administrator Gloria R. Smith, "black nurses were accountable to black people in a special way."[56] As late as 1971, Smith observed that the black nurses would always serve as "spokesmen who could articulate the needs of the black community for compatible care delivery systems as well as the dreams of black people for equal access to and mobility within the health care system."[57] In 1971 black nurses found it desirable again to organize in a separate body to continue the fight for full participation and equal access to opportunities in the profession. The new National Black Nurses' Association reminds us of the resiliency of negative images, racism, discrimination, and the will to overcome injustices of all kinds.

Notes

1. Mary Elizabeth Carnegie, "The Path We Tread," *International Nursing Review* 9 (September–October 1962): 26.
2. Ibid.
3. Ibid.

4. Ibid.

5. Ibid.

6. Joyce Ann Elmore, "Black Nurses: Their Service and Their Struggle," *American Journal of Nursing* 76 (March 1976): 435–37.

7. Jean Maddern Pitrone, *Trailblazer: Negro Nurse in the American Red Cross* (New York: Harcourt, Brace & World, 1969), 88.

8. Ibid., 69.

9. Darlene Clark Hine, "Mable K. Staupers and the Integration of Black Nurses into the Armed Forces," in *Black Leaders of the Twentieth Century,* ed. John Hope Franklin and August Meier (Urbana: University of Illinois Press, 1982), 241–57.

10. Ibid., 254.

11. Philip A. Kalisch and Beatrice J. Kalisch, *The Advance of American Nursing* (Boston: Little, Brown, 1978), 567–68.

12. Quoted in Kalisch and Kalisch, 568.

13. Carter G. Woodson, *The Negro Professional Man in the Community* (New York: Negro Universities Press, [1934] 1969), 142. See chap. 10; the entire chapter, pp. 133–48, is on black nurses.

14. James H. Jones, *Bad Blood: The Tuskegee Syphilis Experiment* (New York: Free Press, 1981), 6.

15. Interview with Eunice Rivers [Laurie], 10 October 1977. Schlesinger Library Black Women's Oral History Project. Radcliffe College, Cambridge, Massachusetts.

16. Ibid.

17. Janet Wilson James, "Isabel Hampton and the Professionalization of Nursing in the 1890s," in *The Therapeutic Revolution: Essays in the Social History of American Medicine,* ed. Morris J. Vogel and Charles E. Rosenberg (Philadelphia: University of Pennsylvania Press, 1979), 201–44; and Celia Davies, "Professionalizing Strategies as Time- and Culture-Bound: American and British Nursing, Circa 1893," in *Nursing History: New Perspectives, New Possibilities,* ed. Ellen Condliffe Lagemann (New York: Teachers College Press, 1983), 47–63.

18. Darlene Clark Hine, "From Hospital to College: Black Nurse Leaders and the Rise of Collegiate Nursing Schools," *Journal of Negro Education* 51 (Summer 1982): 224; George M. Fredrickson, *The Black Image in the White Mind: The Debate on Afro-American Character and Destiny, 1817–1914* (New York: Harper Torchbooks, 1971), 1–179ff; and Anna B. Coles, "The Howard University School of Nursing in Historical Perspective," *Journal of the National Medical Association* 61 (March 1969): 105–18.

19. Sheila Rothman, "Women's Special Sphere," in *Women and the Politics of Culture: Studies in the Sexual Economy,* ed. Michele Wender Zak and Patricia P. Moots (New York: Longman, 1983), 213–23; and Mary Beth Norton, "The Paradox of 'Women's Sphere,'" in *Women of America: A History,* ed. Carol Ruth Berkin and Mary Beth Norton (Boston: Houghton Mifflin, 1979), 139–49.

20. James, 205.

21. Ibid., 203–5.
22. Hine, "From Hospital to College," 224.
23. Daniel H. Williams, "The Need of Hospitals and Training Schools for the Colored People of the South," *National Hospital Record* 3 (April 1900): 3–7; and Booker T. Washington, "Training Colored Nurses at Tuskegee," *American Journal of Nursing* 11 (December 1910): 167–71.
24. Williams, 5.
25. Ibid.
26. Ibid.
27. Ibid., 5–7.
28. Washington, 171.
29. Ibid.
30. John A. Kenney, "Some Facts Concerning Negro Nurse Training Schools and Their Graduates," *Journal of the National Medical Association* 11 (April–June 1919): 53.
31. Ibid.
32. Ethel Johns, "A Study of the Present Status of the Negro Woman in Nursing, 1925" (Unpublished report, 43 pages of typescript plus 16 exhibits, Rockefeller Foundation Archives, Record Group 1.1, Series 200, Box 122, Folder 1507, Rockefeller Archive Center, Pocantico Hills, North Tarrytown, New York 10591-1598), 27.
33. Ibid.
34. Estelle Massey Riddle, "Sources of Supply of Negro Health Personnel: Nurses," *Journal of Negro Education* 6 (Yearbook Issue 1937): 483–92; Johns, 26–27; Darlene Clark Hine, "The Ethel Johns Report: Black Women in the Nursing Profession, 1925," *Journal of Negro History* 67 (Fall 1982): 212–28; and Donelda Hamlin, "Report on Informal Study of the Educational Facilities for Colored Nurses and Their Use in Hospital, Visiting and Public Health Nursing," The Hospital Library and Service Bureau, 1924–25. A copy can be found in Rockefeller Archive Center.
35. Johns, 25.
36. Ibid.
37. Ibid., 29.
38. Ibid., 30.
39. Ibid.
40. Ibid.
41. Ibid, 33.
42. Anna DeCosta Banks, "The Work of a Small Hospital and Training School in the South," *Eighth Annual Report of the Hampton Training School for Nurses and Dixie Hospital* (Hampton, Va.: Hampton Training School for Nurses and Dixie Hospital, 1898–1899): 23–28.
43. Interview with Eunice Rivers [Laurie].
44. James H. Jones, 160.
45. Ibid., 164–67.
46. Elizabeth Jones, "The Negro Woman in the Nursing Profession," *Messenger* 5 (July 1923): 764.

47. Ibid.
48. Pitrone, 99–102; and Coles, 111.
49. W. Montague Cobb, "Mabel Keaton Staupers, R.N., 1890–   ," *Journal of the National Medical Association* 69 (March 1969): 198–99.
50. Mabel Keaton Staupers, "History of the National Association of Colored Graduate Nurses," *American Journal of Nursing* 51 (April 1951): 221–22; and Mabel Keaton Staupers, *No Time for Prejudice* (New York: Macmillan, 1961).
51. Hine, "From Hospital to College," 232.
52. Carnegie, 32.
53. Ibid.
54. Ibid.
55. Ibid., 33.
56. Gloria R. Smith, "From Invisibility to Blackness: The Story of the National Black Nurses' Association," *Nursing Outlook* 23 (April 1975): 226.
57. Ibid.

Janet Muff

9. Of Images and Ideals: A Look at Socialization and Sexism in Nursing

Most nurses are women.[1] The issues that concern nurses are women's is-sues (and vice versa). The problems facing nursing—lack of autonomy, role confusion, disunity, stress, job dissatisfaction, and high turnover—are related to the fact that nursing is a traditionally "woman's job" in a tradi-tionally "man's world." Despite the progress of the women's movement, change is slow. In this chapter I address the traditional and historical prob-lems of nursing, not with the idea that "traditionalism" is of itself good or bad, but that it has meant limited choices for women and nurses.

Nursing identity, an amalgamation of personal and professional values that are derived from socialization and life experience, is central to the problems that face nursing. How nurses see themselves colors their per-ceptions of events, determines their actions, and makes them particularly vulnerable to the damaging effects of sexism and discrimination in the male-dominated health care system. The dual socialization of female nurses—as women and as nurses—to traditional "feminine" identifications contributes to the status and power inequities in nursing.

The key word here is "contributes," because female socialization is not entirely responsible for the current difficulties of nursing. Nurses, them-selves, are responsible. While this may sound a bit like "blaming the vic-tim," it is not. Since publication of my book on women's issues in nursing,[2] I have traveled around the country and spoken with many nurses about their experiences. I have become increasingly aware of two things: first, that it is not experiences themselves that induce stress, but an indi-vidual nurse's *perception* of events and people involved; and second, that perception influences the nurse's response, which in turn influences the reactions of others.

Nurses (and women for that matter), while recognizing the impact of history and culture, can no longer afford to blame others for their problems, but must assume personal responsibility for themselves and their relationships. If there has been any change in my thinking on the subject, it has been a change of focus: from without nursing to within.

Image and Identity: The Impact of Social and Political Forces on Nurses and Nursing

Nursing is stressful. The nature of the job, organizational issues, and interpersonal conflicts are readily apparent sources of stress.[3] Less easy to identify and more insidious in their effects are the antecedents of these stressors, socialization and discrimination.

NURSING: THE IDEAL WORK FOR WOMEN

Women who enter nursing, having been raised in a male-dominated society, usually hold traditional values and attitudes. Traits such as dependence, passivity, and the need for approval unconsciously restrict their options in life to family roles and certain "female" professions.

Historically, occupations have been sex-typed with female occupations being those that developed the "natural," "womanly" attributes of caretaking and housekeeping. Young girls have been channeled into nursing because nursing, in particular, has been seen as good preparation for marriage and motherhood. One might note that it is not nursing that is being sold here, but family life. Through such propaganda, society maintains the status quo.

FEMALE SEX-ROLE SOCIALIZATION.

What is the first question asked when someone has a baby? "Is it a girl or a boy?" Knowing the child's sex is prerequisite, it seems, to responding appropriately. It allows one to activate the correct, preprogrammed series of attitudes and behaviors: pink blankets, fuzzy rabbits, and gentle coos for girls; blue blankets, college trust funds, and tosses in the air for boys. Through such simple, automatic actions, the wheels of destiny are set in motion. From the moment they are born, males and females are treated differently. Little girls learn to be "feminine," meaning passive, dependent, affectionate, emotional, and expressive. They learn that beauty and charm make one desirable to men, and that catching a man is the primary goal. Caring for him and his children is life's work. They learn, too, that the female role is less active, often less enjoyable, and certainly less valued than is the male role.

Children come to think of certain jobs—nursing, teaching, waitressing—as women's work, stopgaps to matrimony. Rarely are girls encouraged to aspire to male-dominated professions. Rarely do they think in terms of lifelong careers. Little boys learn that they will grow up to be policemen, firemen, doctors, lawyers, scientists, and presidents of the United States. Little girls learn that they will grow up to be wives and mommies. If they must work, they may become nurses, or schoolteachers, or waitresses (which are almost like being wives and mommies). The process has been circular. Mothers, themselves members of society, pass on societal values and roles to their daughters. Thus, women are restricted from developing their full human potential by the limited options available to them.

PROFESSIONAL SOCIALIZATION. Traditionally, students enter nursing for nurturant reasons: they want to help people![4] They are, more often than not, well-trained females. Compared with their non-nursing contemporaries, nursing students rate higher on scales measuring dependence, compliance, and submissiveness. Several hypotheses have been formulated as to why this occurs: Guidance counselors and the vocational literature present uninformed and stereotypic pictures of nursing that might channel particularly dependent females into the profession.[5] Perhaps there is something in the recruitment and selection process of nursing schools that attracts such individuals.[6] Youth may play a part. (Nursing students, often new high school graduates, are younger than a random selection of college students.) Whatever the reasons, nursing schools not only admit traditionally oriented women, but also continue to foster such traits through isolationism, authoritarianism, and perfectionism.

Isolationism. Historically, nursing schools have been physically removed from the educational mainstream. As extensions of hospitals, diploma programs fostered apprenticeship learning, frequently under the tutelage of staff physicians. The situation was incestuous and isolating. Even with the move to university-based baccalaureate programs, nursing students continue to demand special (less rigorous) science courses. Such short-sighted practices further isolate nursing students, reduce their credibility, and undermine professional parity. In addition, many attempts by faculty to "professionalize" nursing through the development of nursing models have alienated nurses from each other and from co-workers. This is not to deny the need for nursing theory, but to point out that the use of rigid, impractical, and arbitrary models together with imprecise, often egocentric language does nothing to enhance the image of nursing.

Authoritarianism. Young, female nursing students have traditionally been thought to need protection and guidance. Strict curfews and house rules provided the necessary "discipline." Authoritarianism prevailed in diploma programs and still does to some degree in university programs. Nursing instructors often believe that there is one right way to do things— their way! Their ubiquitous presence precludes independent action by students. Despite lip service that nurses should be autonomous professionals, faculty often reward obedience rather than assertiveness.[7] As a result, fledgling nurses rarely develop the inquisitive, risk-taking behaviors necessary for the world of business.

Perfectionism. Perfectionism is the hallmark of authoritarian faculty. Students in nurses' *training* routinely practice their tasks until perfect. Even the safest, most mundane chores are supervised. Small details are invested with undue significance and danger. Nurses have long been impressed with the "life-or-death" nature of their work, much of which is, in fact, boringly routine. When perfection is the goal, insecurity is the rule. Frustration and disappointment are certain.

The seeds of confusion and dissatisfaction are sown in nursing school. Most students, handicapped with traditional feminine backgrounds, are given the conflicting message: learn to be an autonomous professional, but follow the rules unquestioningly. Nothing could be more crazy-making.

NURSING AS AN OUTGROWTH OF WOMEN'S ROLE. The traditional work of nursing—caretaking and housekeeping—mimics the traditional work of women. Hospitals mimic families,[8] with nurses as obedient daughters to administrator daddies, helpful wives to physician husbands, and loving mothers to patient children:

- Is not the . . . nursing administrator who is responsible for, but does not control, her budget similar to . . . a housewife whose husband doles out the weekly household allowance?
- Is not the . . . staff nurse who not only cares for her patient but cleans beds when housekeepers are not available, assumes secretarial duties when the ward secretary is absent, runs to the pharmacy because the delivery system is broken, and catches hell from a physician and hospital administrator for not being at the desk to greet that physician similar to the . . .

supermom who cares for the house, cares for the kids, cares for her husband, cleans, chauffeurs, juggles, and manages, and who catches hell for forgetting to pick up the drycleaning?

- Is not the . . . nurse who is addressed by physicians as "honey" or "Susie" yet who calls them "Doctor" similar to . . . countless secretaries, waitresses, and airline stewardesses who respond to the males in their lives as "Mister," "Sir," or "Captain?" [sic]
- Is not the . . . critical care nurse who can't say "no" and is pressured into working a double shift because "we can't get anyone else and you can't abandon patients" similar to . . . any woman who has ever said "yes" when she meant "no," who has ever been coerced in the name of selflessness or duty into doing more or giving more than she is able?[9]

Historically, nursing has capitalized on natural "female" traits and has required little formal education. Like other "female" occupations, it has low status, is low paying, and is generally subordinate to men. The role of nursing, like the domestic "female" role, is often unstructured and invisible. Achievements are difficult to define. How, for example, does one *measure* the effects (or the efficacy) of nurturing? To be valued, one must demonstrate value given; yet nurses, like hard-working, obedient daughters, have trusted naively that daddy would notice a job "well done" and reward them. They have been disappointed.

FROM IMAGE TO IDENTITY: DEVELOPMENTAL CONFLICTS IN NURSING

A psychological framework is useful in examining certain identity issues. Most people, both men and women, struggle throughout their lives with basic developmental conflicts: identity and boundary difficulties, dependence-independence issues, problems of self-esteem, greed, and envy. Women are not infantile, nor is there anything innately wrong with them; yet studies indicate that women are, as a group, more dependent, less assertive, and have lower self-esteem than men.[10] The fact is that women have been socialized to these behaviors and difficulties. Nursing continues to struggle with problems of identity and role confusion. These can be examined psychodynamically, *not* as pathological processes, but as developmental milestones. Narcissism and nightingalism, for example, can be healthy or unhealthy, depending on whether they enhance or detract from a person's sense of well-being, relationships with others, and ability to work.

IDENTITY AND BOUNDARY DIFFICULTIES. The child's first task is to begin to differentiate self from other, to develop boundaries, and through this process to learn what is self and what is not self. Nursing, as a profession, is engaged in the same process. Nurses ask themselves: What is nursing and what is not nursing? Where are the boundaries between medicine and nursing? Social work and nursing? Where are the overlaps? What constitutes a professional nurse?

In an effort to answer these questions, some nursing leaders have created false boundaries—arbitrary, alienating models of nursing practice—strongly resisted by practitioners for their lack of clinical applicability. Re-labeling the problem-solving process, for example, and calling it the "nursing" process is an exercise in creative writing rather than theory building. The focus of nursing theoreticians such as these seems egocentric and chauvinistic. Some other leaders now think that to be professional, nursing need not necessarily have a unique body of knowledge and a different language; rather, it must contribute to a shared body of knowledge through *research* and must *use* that body of knowledge in a unique way.[11]

The boundary and identity difficulties of nursing have been reflected historically in problems of giving and receiving. Nurses have, at various times, given away major responsibility for nursing care to non-nurses[12] and taken on the discarded responsibilities of others.[13] The role of nursing has altered in response to the needs of others without conscious decisions by nurses to make those changes. As medicine has become increasingly technical, for example, nurses have assumed many of the tasks previously within the physician's domain. Often, they have been eager to do so, rarely questioning whether such tasks enhanced nursing. More commonly in day-to-day experience, nurses routinely perform housekeeping, secretarial, dietary, and transportation chores when hospitals fail to supply such services, or when those employees are ill. These are all boundary issues involving the delegation of nursing functions to non-nurses, and the performance of non-nursing ones by nurses.

THE DEPENDENCE-INDEPENDENCE BIND. Once a child begins to recognize the difference between self and nonself, her or his next task is to separate and develop greater autonomy. Naturally, conflict arises as the child's quest for independence and mastery is tempered by the external limits imposed by parent and environment. Through trial and error, she or he learns what can and cannot be done; what is "good" and "bad." "Goodness" and "badness," then, are correlated with parental approval.

.

How one sees oneself as an adult, one's sense of self-worth, is also derived in part from the reactions of others. Females grow up defining themselves through their relationships (as someone's daughter, someone's wife, someone's mother), while males define themselves through their actions. Being for others is a large part of traditional female identity; thus, women are more reliant upon others for self-esteem than are men.[14] The *need to be for others,* the reliance on others for self-esteem, makes separation and independence more difficult for women.

Most nurses, as women, experience personal dependence-independence conflicts that are compounded by the authoritarianism of nursing education and the paternalism of typical hospital environments. Many describe problems with assertion—difficulty handling anger and criticism (their own and others'), and difficulty getting their needs met.[15] Some nurses find their confidence easily undermined and have difficulty remembering previous successes with anxiety-laden situations in the face of current anxieties. Their self-esteem is vulnerable.

As a result of the women's movement, most nurses have learned that they *should* be autonomous and assertive. Many chafe at traditional restrictions, yet feel powerless to change their situations. At times, their powerlessness is a perceptual distortion born of prior disappointments. (Too often it is real.) Yet it is the *sense* of powerlessness that makes assertion impossible. Instead of acting on their own behalf, these nurses, caught in seemingly hopelsss situations, often become depressed, angry, or apathetic. They may job hop, burn out, or drop out.

PROBLEMS OF SELF-ESTEEM: NIGHTINGALISM AND NARCISSISM. Young children are narcissistic in that they are self-absorbed. They see people as existing only in relation to themselves; they interpret events in fantastic (from "fantasy") and unrealistic ways. Growing up means giving up infantile narcissism (or seeing things one's own way) for realism (or seeing things as they are). Thus, the child develops a realistic self-concept together with a realistic concept of others.

Self-concept and self-esteem are reciprocal. Through interactions with parents, a child develops a mental image of self to which she or he integrates feelings of "goodness" or "badness" (self-esteem). In this process, a mature sense of self and worth replaces the earlier grandiosity of infantile narcissism. The child develops realistic mental images of others as separate from self and, at the same time, she or he learns to value and care for others. This balance between valuing self, valuing others, and valuing separateness is essential to the capacity for successful relationships.

Problems of identity and self-esteem, when they occur, usually arise in early childhood. Reality may be so painful and/or parental approval so lacking that a child is unable to develop a healthy sense of self. To avoid parental disapproval with its sense of "badness," she or he may present a false, compliant self, outwardly behaving as expected, yet inwardly remaining doubtful of self-worth. To produce the missing sense of "goodness," she or he may cling to the false grandiosity of infantile narcissism.

In a society that values males more, growing up female may be painful. Female socialization encourages selflessness. Approval, hence feelings of self-worth, come from putting others first and oneself last. How can one be self-*less,* and still feel good about one's "self"? Having integrated self-lessness into one's self-concept, how can one develop healthy narcissism (self-esteem)? Females, caught in this double-bind from early childhood, both capitulate and compensate. Outwardly they may present a false, compliant, socially acceptable self while internally preserving unresolved conflicts around issues of self-esteem.

Often, we hear that women are selfless and, less often, that they are narcissistic (except in the superficial, vain sense of the word). The nursing literature discusses many aspects of nightingalism, but only alludes to narcissism. These are not separate entities, but opposite sides of the same coin. Both are present in nursing, although nightingalism is more apparent because it incorporates the dependent, self-sacrificing behaviors to which females have traditionally been socialized, and for which they gain approval.

Nightingalism. Nightingalism is selflessness in nursing parlance. It involves *undervaluing self* and *overvaluing others.* Most nurses enter nursing because they want to help others. They are "trained" to selflessness; they learn to care for others at the expense of themselves. Often, they are seduced or coerced into giving or doing more than they are able in the name of "duty" or "obligation." And the cost is high: guilt if they refuse, resentment if they submit.

Many nurses cannot express their feelings openly and directly because of the power inequities between nursing and hospital administration. Instead, they respond with indirect power plays, passive aggressiveness, and resistance. These behaviors, while sometimes effective over the short term, fail to enhance the image of nurses as powerful, competent professionals.[16]

Narcissism. Healthy narcissism involves caring for oneself; pathological narcissism involves *overvaluing self* and *undervaluing others*. While this is less often recognized among nurses than nightingalism, it exists. The victim or martyr (nightingale), compensating for feelings of anger and powerlessness, often sees her or his sacrifice as enobling and feels superior (narcissist). Such inflated feelings, however, offer false security and are easily shattered.

Nursing has created myths about the role of nurses as helping professionals that, while they bolster narcissism, create undue stress in terms of unrealistic expectations:

- *A "good" nurse cares for all patients equally and is concerned about people all of the time. . . .*
- *A nurse's worth, whether or not she does a "good" job, is related to patient compliance, patient outcome, patient improvement, and patient happiness. . . .*
- *Total patient care means solving all the problems of a patient's whole life: finding him a job, putting a roof over her head, providing food for the table, curing his pain, making her life meaningful, saving their relationships, and so on. . . .*
- *Patients can make us mad, happy, guilty, irritated, and so on.* [While we can trigger emotions in others, they, alone, are responsible for those emotions.] . . .
- *Being a role model means offering oneself as an example of normalcy; being an expert means judging what is right and wrong. . . .*
- *Patients and supervisors and co-workers should appreciate us and our work. . . .*[17]

Such self-glorifying beliefs are narcissistic as well as unrealistic and keep nurses disappointed and frustrated, and encourage power struggles between them and their patients. Studies have shown that nurses can more easily accept powerlessness over the human condition (for example, the patient who dies) than powerlessness over people.[18] Together with the authoritarian, perfectionistic idea that there is only one right way to do things, unhealthy narcissism encourages nurses to "strive to become 'super nurses'—error-free care givers who can do anything."[19] Such attitudes are stressful and make nurses vulnerable to narcissistic injury. Their "self," their worth, is always on the line.

GREED AND ENVY. The transition from dependent, egocentric infant to separating toddler generally occurs in the context of parental love and guidance. Growing self-awareness goes hand-in-hand with growing awareness of others. As a child gains a sense of self and worth, she or he learns to respect others and have concern for them. Greed and envy, primitive emotions that reflect infantile, narcissistic self-absorption, are gradually transformed into less destructive forces by the child's emerging capacity to consider the needs of others.

Greed is insatiable wanting. Envy is wanting that which belongs to another. Both imply no sense of self, no recognition of other as separate from self. "What's mine is mine, and what's yours is mine" expresses the sentiment exactly. Envy destroys what it cannot have. (Jealousy, although derived from envy, is different in several important ways: the jealous person wishes to have what belongs to another, but does not wrest it from the other with brute force, nor destroy it if it cannot be gotten. Jealousy is less primitive than envy because it implies concern for the other.)

Envy and jealousy are fairly common among nurses. The diploma nurse, *envious* of her baccalaureate colleagues, votes against proposals to upgrade nursing educational requirements in her hospital, while another diploma nurse, *jealous* of her baccalaureate colleagues, returns to school to obtain for herself that which they have. The powerless staff nurse, *envious* of her counterparts from temporary agencies who control their own time and earn more money than she does, treats them with contempt and gives them the roughest assignments, making certain they pay for their "ill-gotten" gains. The *jealous* staff nurse, on the other hand, learns from the situation that nurses need not be powerless and identifies strategies for acquiring power herself.

These two components of envy—a sense of entitlement and destructiveness—lie at the root of many nursing conflicts. Take, for example, the case of a psychiatric nurse who developed a weekly women's group for patients. Rather than applauding and supporting her initiative or identifying other patient needs and developing their own groups, her colleagues begrudged her the time, undermined the group, and deplored her "special consideration" to the head nurse.

Unfortunately, the nurse who stands up for her own rights is often envied by her less assertive co-workers, as in the case of a nurse who refused to take voluntary time off during low census periods because she could not afford the loss of income. Other nurses, resentful that they felt obliged to do so, focused their displeasure on her in an attempt to force her capitulation. In yet another hospital where nurses agreed to pool their productivity points and purchase a unit microwave, one nurse declined because she had recently been widowed and needed her points to buy Christmas gifts for her children. In this case, even the head nurse brought pressure to bear, belittling her for lack of "team spirit."

Such experiences are painful and induce fear. Fear of envy leads to defenses that are nondisclosing and isolating, the goal of which is to present oneself in ways that avoid inspiring envy in others. The conscious principle underlying such behaviors is "What they don't know won't hurt them"; the unconscious one is "What they don't know won't hurt *me*." To this end nurses conceal positive aspects of themselves and their practice. For example, a nurse may hesitate to reveal to her colleagues that she is seeking a promotion for fear that they will disparage her ambitions. Baccalaureate nurses, fearing envy, often downplay (and may even deny) the differences between themselves and diploma- or associate-prepared graduates. In this way, fear of envy serves as a real barrier to openness and communication among nurses.

SEXISM AND DISCRIMINATION: PERPETUATING THE IMAGE

"The study of nursing's development in the United States," said Jo Ann Ashley, "is a study of overwhelming obstacles and lack of progress, of discrimination and exploitation."[20] Propaganda about women and work, paternalism from men in medical or administrative hierarchies, and media myths and stereotypes are all forms of discrimination that compound nurses' identity and esteem problems. Studies of job dissatisfaction among nurses indicate that the negative attitudes of others toward and about nursing contribute in large measure to nurses' sense of alienation and powerlessness.

ANATOMY = DESTINY. Woman's place is in the home because women's biology has been used, as propaganda, to keep her there. Caretaking and domestic functions have been designated the special province of females because they involve traditional feminine qualities such as nurturing and a predilection for housework. Despite research that most "feminine" and "masculine" characteristics are learned rather than genetic,[21] the myths and propaganda persist. Women, believing the myths, struggle with conflict and guilt over assuming nontraditional roles and limiting or abandoning traditional ones.

Nursing, as a caricature of femininity, is subject to the same discrimination as are females in general. In the same way that women's work has often been devalued, the work of nurses is devalued as "natural" rather than learned, and as "art" rather than science. Sexist thinking about nursing hypothesizes that because nursing is not an intellectual discipline, nurses need not receive higher education; apprenticeship learning is sufficient. Because nursing requires no special skills, anyone (any woman) can do it. Because it involves caretaking and domestic functions, it is ideal preparation for marriage. Because the practice of nursing comes "naturally" to women, they can return to it easily after many years' hiatus.

The goal of such propaganda is to maintain the status quo, to keep nurses "barefoot, pregnant, and in the kitchen." And it works. Nurses, themselves, repudiate the need for advanced education. Often they believe that a-nurse-is-a-nurse-is-a-nurse, and that all nurses have the same (natural) skills and should be able to work anywhere. High turnover and drop-out rates indicate that many nurses do not see nursing as a lifelong career, but as a "stopgap to marriage" or "something to fall back on."[22] But perhaps the most significant effect of sexual discrimination is economic: if nursing is natural, requires little education and few special skills, then it is not worth much and need not be remunerated.

PATERNALISM AND INSTITUTIONALIZED POWERLESSNESS. Historically, women's work and contributions to society have been demeaned by those who jokingly asked, "What were women doing while men created masterpieces?" The answer has long been obvious to women: they were raising, feeding, protecting, serving, supporting, and freeing up the men who were creating masterpieces. *And* they were creating masterpieces in their own right—intricate, marvelously artistic quilts, samplers, and embroideries, for example—which were devalued as "crafts" rather than true art because of their unconventional medium.

Women, and nurses, concealed in the wings, have always served the men in their lives, benefiting vicariously through their successes. Women's work has been secondary and subservient to men's work. In health care, physicians have done the curing, using intellectual, scientific skills, while nurses have done the caring, using their "natural female" attributes. Curing has been valued and recompensed; caring has not. Nurses, themselves failing to recognize and value that which they do, have continued to work, trusting that others (physicians and administrators) would recognize and reward them.

The power inequities between medicine and nursing have been institutionalized in settings where physicians report directly to the board of directors while nurses report through administration. Despite the fact that nursing departments generally have the most employees and the greatest responsibility for patient care, they generally do *not* have direct access to the governing bodies of their facilities.

The contributions of nursing go unrecognized largely because physicians are seen as the primary care providers and because nursing is seen as an economic drain. In a health care system where laboratory tests and even surgery can be performed on an outpatient basis, the only reasons a person need be hospitalized is to receive nursing care. Yet nursing services are commonly lumped together with housekeeping, dietary, and maintenance charges as part of the basic "room rate."

Naturally, the revenue generated by various departments determines their share of the budget. Because nurses do not routinely bill for services, they are handicapped in the competition for personnel and resources. At a time when fiscal responsibility is crucial to survival, nursing is seen as an economic liability rather than an asset. Thus, nursing's lack of control over practice stems from failure of access and failure to demonstrate revenue produced. These two factors, as direct results of paternalism and discrimination, perpetuate the powerlessness from which they sprang.

PROPAGANDA. Propaganda inevitably uses some aspect of its target—socialization, personality traits, situational power inequities—to unfair advantage. Traditional female socialization, the earliest form of propaganda, is effective because even the oppressed believe what they are taught about themselves. Women pass on societal values to their daughters. Nurses, as targets of propaganda designed to keep them in a dependent, second-class status, accept or are confused by what they hear, but rarely repudiate it. Often they do not recognize what is happening, that they are being manipulated, because the process is covert.

Nurses' strivings for professionalism, for example, have been exploited by those who would maintain the handmaiden image. To this end nurses are told that uniforms are "professional"—as are caps. Yet nurses rarely point out that it is service workers, not professionals, who wear uniforms. And when asked to work a double shift, they are told that "patients need you and we can't get anyone else." Carrying charts on rounds with physicians is also *very* professional. Despite growing resentment over the doctor-nurse game, nurses may have difficulty abandoning traditional rituals like making chart rounds, because to do so might mean conflict and the work of developing whole new ways of relating with physicians. Yet, as Venner Farley so aptly says, "if nurses were meant to be portable chart racks, they would have been born with wheels."[23] Altruism and selflessness are so deeply ingrained through female socialization that to refuse a patient's needs, no matter how logical the grounds, is to experience guilt.

Flattery is a particularly destructive form of propaganda used to divide and conquer. Day nurses, for example, are told that they are so much more skilled than night nurses, and they believe it. Critical care nurses are told that they are better nurses than their med-surg counterparts, and they, too, believe it. What many nurses fail to recognize is that flattery is most likely some form of manipulation. The flatterer undoubtedly wants something, and uses the nurses' own narcissism to get it. Comparisons with other nurses are used to drive a wedge. Statements like "You're always so responsible, I knew I could count on you" are often used to lower resistance and make refusal difficult.

Historically, nurses have been paid less than they are worth, and certainly less than traditionally masculine occupations of similar education and responsibility. Discrimination and propaganda have kept nurses' salaries artificially low in a determined effort to maintain the status quo. Nursing, as we know, defies the traditional laws of supply and demand.[24] Theoretically, in a free economy, a "shortage" of nurses should cause their salaries to rise dramatically, reflecting nurses' high market value. That has not occurred because, in actuality, the economy has not been "free." Unbeknownst to nurses, hospital administrators have met regularly to standardize nursing salaries in their communities.

The nursing "shortage," when it existed, was used as an excuse to lower standards, reduce nursing care hours, and employ ancillary staff to provide nursing services. Believing propaganda that money was in short supply, nurses failed to use their scarcity as leverage. Even while questioning the outpouring of funds for hospital expansions, costly equipment purchases, and perks for physicians, rarely did nurses act on their discontent. The current nursing "surplus," coupled with "economic cut-backs," is being used to achieve similar ends. Fearing for their livelihoods, nurses acquiesce to further reductions in nursing care hours, lower salaries, the loss of twelve-hour shifts, and changes in the nursing delivery system that remove nurses from the bedside and replace them with non-licensed personnel.

MEDIA MYTHS AND STEREOTYPES. Throughout history myths have evolved that tell us that woman is, by nature, an all-loving Madonna and, alternately, an evil seductress. She is angelic and bitchy, nurturing and castrating, the wholesome "girl next door" and a "two-bit tramp." Stereotypic images of nursing caricaturize womanhood and reflect basic human conflicts over good and evil.[25] When one thinks of a "nurse," what images come to mind? A white cap and blue cape? An angel of mercy? A starched spinster? Cool, soothing hands? Rough, probing hands? Medications? Ministrations? Bedbaths? Bedpans? Bed mates? The images are varied depending on one's experience and vantage point.

The media commonly depict six major nursing stereotypes:

Angel of Mercy
Handmaiden to the physician
Woman in white
Sex symbol/idiot
Battle-ax
Torturer[26]

All project the image of nurses as females, and none reflects the intelligence necessary for nursing. Media nurses are more often diploma than associate or baccalaureate degree graduates despite the decline in hospital schools. Whether in books, magazines, television, or movies, nurses are generally portrayed in traditional, even obsolete, roles. With the possible exception of nurses in the news, rarely are the specialization, sophistication, and autonomy of nursing communicated by media characters.

The impact of individual articles or programs is negligible. It is the collective impact over time, the cumulative effect, that influences nursing's image in a negative way. Stereotypes generate expectations. People, programmed by the media to think of nurses as angels or handmaidens or torturers, are ill-prepared for real-life nursing. Occasionally they are relieved or disappointed (that nurses are neither so "bad" nor so "good" as they imagined); most often they are confused.

Media stereotypes undoubtedly influence recruitment by presenting inaccurate images of nursing to the uninitiated. Likewise, they influence nursing practice by making it incumbent on nurses to reeducate patients and co-workers as to the real nature of their work. Finally, and indirectly, because they contribute to nursing stress, these negative, inaccurate stereotypes influence nursing retention.

Ideal vs. Reality: Stress and Conflict in Nursing

The issues just discussed—socialization, sexism, and stereotyping—have a fundamental, yet largely unrecognized, impact on nursing. Nurses are overwhelmed, confused, and divided. Perceiving themselves as powerless to change an intolerable situation, they feel trapped and experience stress. Nursing, as a profession, is (and has been for as long as anyone can remember) "at the crossroads" with no apparent sense of direction. Current political and economic trends in health care are changing nursing via the ripple effect, yet rarely are nurses in a shaping position. They are more often reactive than pro-active.[27]

INDIVIDUAL ISSUES

The nursing shortage may be a thing of the past in most parts of this country, but the drop in turnover and vacancy rates should not be interpreted to mean that the problems of nurses in hospitals have been solved or that nurses are happier at their jobs. This is frequently not the case. Many nurses are working out of financial necessity. Trapped by economic constraints and an unfavorable job market, nurses can no longer move freely from job to job. There are fewer escape hatches—no parachutes. The issue of choice, or lack of it, is central to the increasing stress experienced by individual nurses.

In addition, many nurses are faced with professional-bureaucratic role conflict. Hospitals, supposedly in the business of caring for patients, often seem more concerned with attracting physicians and expanding profits. While there is nothing wrong with making money, there *is* something wrong when patients and employees feel mangled by bureaucratic machinery.

Nurses, traditionally naive and altruistic, are shocked and hurt in such situations. Frequently they experience cognitive dissonance over what they believe they *ought* to be doing versus what they are being told to do. Such conflict is too painful to be tolerated for long. Since leaving their jobs is less of an option, nurses must either develop defenses against such feelings (and in so doing become depressed or apathetic) or resolve the conflict in some way. Because it is often easier to change themselves than the situation, resolving the conflict often takes the form of relinquishing nursing values for organizational ones. There are some data to indicate that nurses become less professional after working several years.[28] This may very well be the result of nurses' limited options in the face of painful professional-bureaucratic conflict.

INTERPERSONAL ISSUES

Historically, nursing has been fraught with man-woman problems (paternalism, doctor-nurse games) and woman-woman problems (sibling rivalry, queen bee syndrome). The origins of these conflicts are developmental and societal. Freudian theories tell us that woman hates man because she envies his penis; she hates women because her mother failed to give her a penis. Such explanations seem incomplete because they neglect to take into account the effects of sexual discrimination in a society that favors males. Feminist and sociological theories suggest that if women envy men, it is for their opportunities and freedom and power, and that if women hate women, it is because they have learned self-hate from a culture that molds them into a feminine role and then devalues that role.

NURSE AGAINST NURSE. "Nurses," we hear, "are their own worst enemies." They belittle, poke fun at, and do not respect each other. This phenomenon of like-against-like is described by sociologists as *horizontal violence*.[29] At its most blatant, such conflict among nurses can be seen in the bickering among diploma, associate, and baccalaureate nurses, in the rivalry between shifts, and in the rites of passage for new graduates. At its most subtle, horizontal violence is evident in nurses' reliance on medical rather than nursing consultation, their lack of involvement in professional organizations, and their failure to perceive women's issues and nursing issues as their own.

When the violence is vertical, that is between superiors and subordinates, sociologists call it the *queen bee syndrome*,[30] and psychoanalysts call it *identification with the aggressor*.[31] Nurses, as we know, cannot tolerate powerlessness and pain indefinitely. One solution, identified earlier, is to relinquish nursing values for those of the organization; one way to feel powerful is to align with those who have power. A common example is the nursing director who loses her nursing identity and fails to support the economic and professional progress of her staff.[32]

While horizontal and vertical violence do exist in nursing, they are not the result of biologic deficiencies. Women are not born catty, bitchy, and hateful. Research indicates that members of minority groups commonly develop self-hate and hatred of their own kind.[33] Whereas nurses are not in a numerical minority, they have been discriminated against both as women and as nurses. If they have not learned to value themsleves (because society does not value them), how can they value others like themselves? Given their history, is it any wonder that nurses have difficulty respecting and asserting themselves and respecting and supporting their peers?

PHYSICIAN-NURSE CONFLICT. Much has been written about the conflict between physicians and nurses. Virtually every nurse has tried, in her own way, to solve the problem—yet it continues. Historically, nurses have been dependent on and subservient to physicians just as wives have been dependent on and subservient to husbands. Such power inequities produce pain and anger, and women, despite their socialization to be meek, have certainly experienced the pain and anger, together with their own undaunted strivings for independence. Chafing at and resisting the bonds of convention, they have struggled with the powerful men in their lives for self-determination.

In addition to the "male-female" theory, several hypotheses have been put forward as to the sources of physician-nurse conflict[34]—physicians' lack of understanding of the nurse's role, their antiquated self-image as captain of the ship, their erroneous belief that patients value their services more highly than those of nurses, and nurses' failure to clarify their role and to assert themselves in a professional manner. All are probably valid and contribute to the problem. Recent changes in third-party payment, which give nurses the authority to question (and even refuse) unnecessary tests and procedures ordered by physicians for patients, will undoubtedly make matters worse. The balance of power is shifting, and it will be up to nurses whether or not they make use of the opportunity.

POWER STRUGGLES WITH PATIENTS. Nurses, seeing themselves as advocates, experts, and role models, often find themselves engaged in power struggles with patients. Statements like "he's only doing this for attention," "she's manipulative," and "the doctor took the patient's side" are indicative of such conflicts. They reflect negative value judgments of patients' behavior and illustrate nurses' narcissistic sense of righteousness and omnipotence.

Patients who are described as manipulators and attention seekers often are those who disagree with nurses over what is best for themselves and who engage in getting their needs met, regardless of nurses' opinions. Generally they are quite direct—they telephone physicians, thereby circumventing the nurses, and they use their call lights to great advantage. Such behaviors may be infuriating, but they are not manipulative.

The narcissistic overinvestment of many nurses in their patients makes conflict inevitable and painful. Too often nurses (and other helping professionals) believe that because they may have greater scientific knowledge or clinical expertise, they also have the right to judge patients' behaviors and to expect compliance. That is not the case. Being an advocate or an expert means proffering one's knowledge and services on request, with the understanding that patients may accept or reject them. Yet, because the self-concept of many nurses depends on being allowed to do for others, rejection hurts. And because their self-worth depends on patient compliance, conflict ensues.

PROFESSIONAL ISSUES

Socialization and discrimination adversely affect not only individual nurses, but also the profession as a whole by contributing to role confusion and problems of recruitment and retention. In addition, they perpetuate male domination of health care and the alienation of nurses from each other and women in general.

When one looks at the problems of the nursing role, it soon becomes apparent that nurses are divided into multiple splinter groups, each defining nursing in a different way. One split exists between diploma, associate, and baccalaureate graduates; another lies between nurses in practice and nurses in education; and still other splits occur geographically. It is virtually impossible to arrive at a consensus among nurses on political or philosophical issues (but on one issue—economics—they all agree: nurses are not paid what they are worth).

The problem is not that nurses disagree, but that they allow their lack of agreement to interfere with their work by expending time and energy intellectualizing about philosophical issues, debating and justifying the professional status of nursing, and distinguishing the role of nurses from other health care providers. Such narcissistic investment and defensiveness indicate lack of security. It is as if nurses, because they are not at all sure of themselves and nursing, must continually engage in proving their status and worth. In the words of Shakespeare, they "protest too much."

Lack of unity interferes with nursing progress in another way: it is used as an excuse for not getting the work done. Like a red herring, it focuses attention and energy away from the real problems, thus allowing them to continue. Nursing's failure to solve economic, political, and practice issues, for example, is blamed on lack of unity among nurses. How many times do we hear: "If only nurses would join together (get organized, become cohesive) the problems would be solved"? In essence, it is not unity that nurses desire as much as homogeneity. Their wish, that all nurses would think alike, agree on major issues, and want the same things, stems from the unrealistic belief that a-nurse-is-a-nurse-is-a-nurse (and that all nurses should be like me).

Even when nurses "understand" their role, many have difficulty articulating it. They say, "I know what I'm doing and why, but I can't put it into words." Often they rely on uniforms to define themselves, mistakenly assuming that others, on seeing the uniform, will know that they are nurses and understand what they do. In fact, many occupations—dieticians, technicians, and nursing assistants—wear white uniforms. As to the idea that people understand the nursing role, this is simply not so. If media images of nursing are any indication of public understanding, it is clearly evident that people are not aware of what nurses do.

This lack of public awareness influences both nursing recruitment and retention. How nurses are seen determines the kind of people who enter the profession. The overall stereotype of a white Anglo-Saxon Protestant/Catholic female under thirty eliminates many potential candidates. In addition, nursing no longer has the advantage of a captive audience because the women's movement has opened the doors of traditionally male occupations to females. The best and the brightest are now going elsewhere. Nursing school enrollments have dropped as women, seeking high-status, high-powered, high-paying careers shun the stereotypic image of nursing. And nurses themselves, tired of battling misconceptions, redefining the role, and living up (or down) to unrealistic expectations, often leave nursing.

The continued domination of health care (and nurses) by powerful, traditionally male groups—physicians, hospital administrators, and insurance companies—makes nursing unattractive to contemporary women and men. It not only contributes to stress and conflict in the clinical arena, but also inhibits the progress of nursing education. Despite the move to academic settings, many nursing schools continue to fall under medicine's umbrella. If anything, there is currently a renewed effort by schools of medicine to incorporate schools of nursing.[35]

Whether nursing survives today's economic crisis as a professional discipline will depend largely on nurses' ability not only to weather the storm, but also to take advantage of the power it gives them. Cost consciousness demands that nurses define exactly what it is they do and makes them overseers of patient services. While other disciplines (social work, respiratory therapy, physical therapy) struggle to justify their very existence, nursing is seen by many as a jack-of-all-trades. On the one hand, this may be interpreted as a put-down; on the other hand, as an opportunity. For the first time, nurses are being asked to define their competencies and thereby delineate the boundaries of their profession. In addition, they are being treated as the equals of physicians, as colleagues who, in their capacity as patient advocates, have the power and authority to recommend or refuse treatment.

The ball is in nursing's court, so to speak. To win, nurses must recognize problem areas and do something about them. They must:

1. Recognize women's issues as their issues.
    - Become aware of sexual discrimination in all areas of society: home, school, business, religion, government, etc.
    - Value traditionally "feminine" traits such as compassion, caring, and expressiveness, and combine them with traditionally "masculine" traits such as assertion, independence, and analytic ability, thus becoming androgynous.
    - Refuse to put down other women or to find humor in that which demeans womanhood.
    - Identify sexism in health care, specifically in the areas of obstetrics, gynecology, and psychiatry.
2. Recognize identity problems.
    - Define boundaries and roles (individually and collectively).
    - Articulate boundaries and roles (individually and collectively).
    - Develop a realistic self-image by relinquishing narcissism and victimization.
3. Recognize dependence/independence issues.
    - Identify the seductiveness of being dependent on paternalistic and maternalistic figures.
    - Accept that a cage, even if gilded, is still a cage.
    - Identify the risks and trade-offs of becoming assertive.
    - Accept responsibility for selves no matter how frightening or painful that may be.
    - Get help, if necessary: therapy, consciousness-raising, assertiveness training, networking, support groups, etc.
4. Recognize perceptual distortions.
    - Acknowledge the tendency to interpret events negatively and to see selves as powerless.
    - Abandon pessimism; develop objectivity, even optimism (for example, a kick in the pants by one's boss can be interpreted as "being stepped on" or as a "boost up the ladder to success").

- Learn to "make lemonade out of lemons" by identifying opportunities and choices in difficult situations.

5. Recognize interpersonal difficulties.
- Understand that power is rarely given up without a struggle; expect and learn to handle conflict with physicians when challenging their power.
- Develop tact and negotiating skills.
- Distinguish between rebelliousness and assertion; between defensiveness and assertion.
- Learn to deal with envy and greed.
- Support other nurses; recognize that not everyone can be a leader, but one can always lick stamps, work behind the scenes, etc.
- Encourage and value heterogeneity among nurses.
- Identify potential areas of conflict with patients and deactivate own "buttons."

6. Recognize the need for business acumen.
- Acquire personal power by developing one's image, being visible, learning the ropes, cultivating power sources.
- Acquire professional power by negotiating fees for service, access to governing bodies, voting membership on medical staff committees, admitting privileges, etc.
- Acquire business skills, savvy.

7. Recognize propaganda, stereotypes, sexism.
- Identify own contribution to propaganda, stereotypes, sexism.
- Speak out.
- Write to producers, advertisers, publishers.
- Educate nurses, other professionals, the public.

8. Recognize professional issues.
- Support higher education in nursing.
- Participate in research and theory development.
- Join professional organizations.
- Keep abreast of legislation. Vote.

The time for passivity is over. Emerging trends in health care make active participation by nurses necessary for survival. This, undoubtedly, involves risk—of failure, of rejection, of sanctions—but the rewards are great. The future looks hopeful for nursing *if* nurses will open their eyes, lower their defenses, commit themselves to action, and reach out to each other.

Notes

1. Ninety-six percent of nurses are women. The image of a "nurse" is that of a female. In this paper I will deal with nursing, then, as a female occupation. There are certainly men in nursing. They have problems, even image and identity problems, but the image and identity problems of *nursing* are female.

2. Janet Muff, *Socialization, Sexism, and Stereotyping: Women's Issues in Nursing* (St. Louis: C. V. Mosby, 1982).

3. Janet Muff, "Origins of Stress in Nursing," in *Surviving Nursing*, ed. Emily E. M. Smythe (Menlo Park, Calif: Addison-Wesley, 1984), 13–37.

4. Helen Cohen, "Authoritarianism and Dependency: Problems in Nursing Socialization," in *Current Perspectives in Nursing: Social Issues and Trends*, vol. 2, ed. Beverly C. Flynn and Michael H. Miller (St. Louis: C. V. Mosby, 1980), 160.

5. Denise W. Benton, "You Want To Be a What?" *Nursing Outlook* 27 (June 1979): 388.

6. Myrita K. Flanagan, "An Analysis of Nursing as a Career Choice," in *Socialization, Sexism, and Stereotyping: Women's Issues in Nursing*, ed. Janet Muff (St. Louis: C. V. Mosby, 1982), 169–77.

7. Cohen, 161.

8. Jo Ann Ashley, *Hospitals, Paternalism, and the Role of the Nurse* (New York: Teachers College Press, 1976).

9. Muff, "Origins of Stress," 23.

10. Ella Lasky, "Sources of Feminine Self-Esteem," in *Humanness: An Exploration into the Mythologies about Women and Men*, ed. Ella Lasky (New York: MSS Corporation, 1975), 63–66.

11. Phoebe Hughes McMurrey, "Toward a Unique Knowledge Base in Nursing," *Image* 14 (February/March 1982): 12; and Sherry L. Shamansky and Celeste R. Yanni, "In Opposition to Nursing Diagnosis: A Minority Opinion," *Image* 15 (Spring 1983): 47.

12. Ingeborg Mauksch, "An Analysis of Some Critical Contemporary Issues in Nursing," *Journal of Continuing Education in Nursing* 14 (July/August 1983): 4.

13. Venner Farley, "Power and Politics in Nursing," Lecture presented to the Orange County Nursing Consortium, Golden West College, Huntington Beach, California, September 1983.

14. Lasky, 64.

15. Bonnie W. Duldt, "Helping Nurses Cope with the Anger-Dismay Syndrome," *Nursing Outlook* 30 (March 1982): 168; and Jeffrey A. Kelly, "Sex-Role Stereotypes and Mental Health: Conceptual Models in the 1970s and Issues for the 1980s," in *The Stereotyping of Women: Its Effects on Mental Health*, ed. V. Franks and E. D. Rothblum (New York: Springer, 1983), 11–29.

16. Teddy Langford, "The Nurse Martyr: A Dying Breed," *Nursingworld Digest* (7 June 1982): 20.

17. Muff, "Origins of Stress," 29–30.

18. Ray L. Smith, Gerald Kushel, and Lester Korabow, "Power," *Nursing Life* 2 (July/August 1982): 27.

19. Cohen, 162.

20. Ashley, *Hospitals,* ix.

21. Lenore Weitzman, "Sex-Role Socialization," in *Women: A Feminist Perspective,* ed. Jo Freeman (Palo Alto, Calif.: Mayfield, 1979), 153–216.

22. Linda Hughes, "Little Girls Grow Up To Be Wives and Mommies: Nursing as a Stopgap to Marriage," in *Socialization, Sexism, and Stereotyping: Women's Issues in Nursing,* ed. Janet Muff (St. Louis: C. V. Mosby, 1982), 157–68.

23. Farley.

24. Mauksch, 4.

25. Janet Muff, "Handmaiden, Battle-Ax, Whore: An Exploration into the Fantasies, Myths, and Stereotypes about Nurses," in *Socialization, Sexism, and Stereotyping: Women's Issues in Nursing,* ed. Janet Muff (St. Louis: C. V. Mosby, 1982), 114.

26. Ibid., 120.

27. Laurie Glass and Karen Brand, "The Progress of Women and Nursing: Parallel or Divergent?" in *Women in Stress: A Nursing Perspective,* ed. D. K. Kjervik and I. M. Martinson (New York: Appleton-Century-Crofts, 1979), 31–45.

28. Martha N. Sleicher, "Nursing Is Not a Profession," in *Nursing in Transition,* ed. T. A. Duespohl (Rockville, Md.: Aspen Systems Corporation, 1983), 3–13.

29. Florynce Kennedy, "Institutionalized Oppression *vs.* the Female," in *Sisterhood is Powerful,* ed. Robin Morgan (New York: Vintage Books, 1970), 438–46.

30. G. Staines, C. Tauris, and T. B. Jayarline, "The Queen Bee Syndrome," *Psychology Today* 7 (August 1974): 55.

31. Norman Cameron, *Personality Development and Psychotherapy* (Boston: Houghton-Mifflin, 1963), passim.

32. Mauksch, 5.

33. Helen Mayer Hacker, "Women as a Minority Group," in *Women: A Feminist Perspective,* ed. Jo Freeman (Palo Alto, Calif.: Mayfield, 1979), 505–20.

34. Beatrice J. Kalisch and Philip A. Kalisch, "An Analysis of the Sources of Physician-Nurse Conflict," in *Socialization, Sexism, and Stereotyping: Women's Issues in Nursing,* ed. Janet Muff (St. Louis: C. V. Mosby, 1982), 221–33.

35. Jo Ann Ashley, private communication, Fall 1980.

Anne Hudson Jones

10. *The White Angel* (1936): Hollywood's Image of Florence Nightingale*

Since 1854 the most powerful and influential image of a nurse has been that of the lady with a lamp—Florence Nightingale making her nightly rounds in the Barrack Hospital at Scutari during the Crimean War.[1] Single-handedly, it seems, she changed the image of the nurse from the prevailing one of the ignorant drunken bawd—the Sairey Gamp[2]—to that of the ministering angel. She combined elements of the monastic and military traditions to create such a dramatically improved image of nursing that respectable women of all classes could choose nursing as a secular profession without fear of social disgrace. Nightingale is still referred to as the mother of modern nursing.

The image of Florence Nightingale has been nearly as popular and powerful in the United States as it has been in England. In 1857 the American poet Henry Wadsworth Longfellow immortalized her image as the "lady with a lamp" in his poem "Santa Filomena." This popular image of her was renewed in the United States in 1936 when Warner Brothers released *The White Angel*, the first Hollywood film biography of Florence Nightingale. Warner Brothers had been pleased with the success of their medical biography *The Story of Louis Pasteur*, released earlier in the year. *The White Angel* was to be a feminine follow-up.[3] In speculating about its importance in reinforcing the popular image of Florence Nightingale, we should remember that *The White Angel* was released during a decade when movies dominated American popular culture. Estimates are that during the 1930s, average weekly attendance at the movies was between sixty and ninety million people.[4]

More to the point in assessing the importance for nursing of the image presented in the film, the premiere showing of *The White Angel* on June

*I thank Karen Kingsley and Robert L. Jones for their helpful comments and criticisms.

24, 1936, in Los Angeles, coincided with the Biennial Convention of the American Nurses' Association (ANA), which was also held in Los Angeles. The film's premiere was announced in the June 1936 issue of the *American Journal of Nursing,* which had run two pages of stills from the film in its May 1936 issue.[5] In August 1936, the ANA board of directors announced its formal endorsement of *The White Angel* because the film

> effectively and dramatically shows:
> 1. The importance of selecting young women of education, character, and courage for nursing;
> 2. The necessity for providing for them a sound education in nursing in accordance with the needs of the time.[6]

The board went on to encourage "district, alumnae, or other groups of nurses" to use showings of the film at their local theaters to raise funds for the Florence Nightingale International Foundation.

Also in August 1936, *Public Health Nursing* reviewed *The White Angel* very favorably. While recognizing that "some liberties have been taken with historical facts," the reviewer was pleased that "the story unfolds itself entirely without propaganda."[7] In fact, the reviewer went on to suggest that the film carries a lesson for those in public health nursing who might want to interpret their work to the public. *The White Angel* was held up as a model of "a good educational picture" because it does not use direct propaganda or excessive technical detail. The reviewer closed: "We commend this picture to the thoughtful consideration of laymen as well as nurses, especially those concerned with education and information."[8]

General reviews of *The White Angel* were less enthusiastic than those of organized nursing, but they also stressed the important educational aspect of the film. For example, in its June 1936 issue, *Variety* suggested that it was a mistake to release the picture in June, when schools were just out, because schools would have produced an organized attempt to get students to see the film. The reviewer thought the film's major appeal would be educational, and he suggested that *The White Angel* would need tie-ups with medical and hospital groups if it were to do well at the box office. The *New York Times* reviewer praised the film for having only minor historical infidelities, but found fault with its editorializing of the heroine's life, saying that she is presented as a historical character rather than as a real person. The general reviewers proved to be right. The film never achieved the success that many other films of the 1930s attained, but it is a fascinating educational effort. That it was perceived and publicized as such, and formally endorsed by the ANA, makes its image of Florence Nightingale all the more important.

In fact, the qualities that make Florence Nightingale historically significant are not those usually associated with a good nurse. Nor are they the qualities most emphasized in *The White Angel*. Nightingale succeeded because she was a tough-minded pragmatist, an organizational and administrative genius, a political schemer, a powerfully assertive woman, and a troublemaker. To make her image palatable for a popular audience *The White Angel* tailors her qualities to fit the prevailing patterns of the 1930s. Despite the 1930s trappings, however, the archetypal images of nurse as mother, seductress, and nun emerge iconographically as the most powerful in the film.

The White Angel credits Mordaunt Shairp with the screenplay; reviews and reference books credit Lytton Strachey's 1918 biographical essay on Florence Nightinagle, from his book *Eminent Victorians,* as the basis for the film.[9] Although Strachey based his essay on the excellent, standard two-volume biography of Florence Nightingale published by Sir Edward Cook in 1913, Strachey's purpose was quite different from Cook's. Whereas Cook wrote a 1,017-page highly detailed yet tactful biography, Strachey wrote a 68-page character sketch designed to expose the true Florence Nightingale and debunk the popular notion of her. He considered her to be demon-possessed: at the same time, more interesting and less likable than the popular image of her.[10] Ironically, given the credits, *The White Angel* disregards Strachey's purpose and tone and reinstates the familiar, popularized version of Nightingale as the saintly, self-sacrificing woman, the legendary lady with a lamp.

Nonetheless, the screenplay for *The White Angel* was carefully, even impressively, researched. There is a factual basis for almost everything in the film. Often, however, the facts have been altered in ways that reduce Nightingale from Strachey's powerful, albeit demonic, image of her to the more popular and palatable one. It is fascinating, especially in light of the film's perceived educational value, to analyze these alterations and contrast Hollywood's image of Florence Nightingale with the image of Nightingale presented in earlier biographies and histories. Examining the alterations and the iconography of this film helps highlight the most significant ingredients of the popular image that Hollywood's Nightingale bequeathed to her professional descendants.

Many of the film's changes result from condensing Nightingale's long life (1820–1910) to fit the constraints of a 75-minute feature film. The first way of doing this was to focus only on Nightingale's best known experiences, those of the Crimean War: the film begins at midnight on New Year's Day 1850 and ends in the summer of 1856, with Nightingale's audience with Queen Victoria. This condensation of time creates a fundamental distortion. For example, one of the early episodes from Nightingale's life that is almost always mentioned by biographers is her treating the wounded leg of a dog named Cap. This episode is popular because it seems an early portent of Nightingale's later career. Strachey mentions this episode only in passing.[11] In his biography, Cook gives the episode in more detail, basing his account on a letter to Nightingale from her old pastor, the Reverend J. T. Giffard. According to Giffard's letter, the episode took place in 1836 on the downs near Embley, the Nightingale country estate. Shepherd Smithers had planned to hang his collie, Cap, to put it out of its misery from a hurt leg; Nightingale's successful treatment of the dog saved its life.[12] Nightingale was sixteen years old at the time.

This episode with Cap is included in *The White Angel*, but in a considerably revised fashion. That the screenwriter had this same episode in mind is evidenced by the dog's name, Cap. In the film, the incident occurs in 1850 in London, when Nightingale would have been thirty years old. While she is playing the piano to entertain her suitor, Charles, she hears Cap yelping and barking. Florence and Charles rush out to find that a carriage has run over Cap and broken his leg. Florence picks up Cap, carries him into the library, and expertly splints his leg. Mr. Sidney Herbert, who has just arrived with his wife, assists Florence and assures Charles that there is no need to call a doctor since Florence is there.

These changes affect the whole quality of the incident. Nightingale, shown in her Victorian finery, attends a small lap dog in the library of a fashionable London residence, with Charles and her soon-to-be advisor and comrade Sidney Herbert in attendance. Making Cap a pet, a small lap dog rather than a shepherd's working dog; moving the incident from the countryside at Embley to the city of London; and using the incident to characterize a thirty-year-old instead of a sixteen-year-old all trivialize the episode. It no longer serves the same purpose it did in earlier biographies: to show how early the inclination to nursing manifested itself in Nightingale's behavior. In the film it foreshadows Nightingale's decision to become a nurse, but does so only a few scenes before Nightingale announces her decision.

We know from Strachey and Cook that Nightingale had struggled for many years to find useful work for herself and to be allowed to become a nurse, an occupation considered unfitting for an educated, affluent Victo-

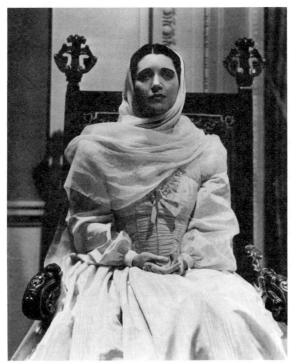

FIGURE 10-1. Kay Francis as Florence Nightingale in white. *The White Angel.* Copyright © 1936 Warner Bros. Pictures, Inc. Renewed 1963 United Artists Associated, Inc. Photo courtesy Academy of Motion Pictures Arts and Sciences. Reproduced with permission of Turner Entertainment Co.

rian lady. In the film, her decision to become a nurse is instantaneous, a result of her having read one of her father's reports on the conditions of hospitals in London. In a dramatic scene, she confronts her mother and father and sister as they return from a dinner party one evening, and she emphatically announces to them that she has decided to become a nurse. Her decision is as sudden and forceful as a religious conversion.

In this scene she is dressed in white, thus visually fulfilling the image of the title (Fig. 10-1), but the image does more than just show Nightingale in white. Her dress and veil are like a bridal gown and veil in style as well as color. The association of white with virginity and purity is important, as is the bridal association. At the same time she announces her decision to be a nurse, Nightingale announces to her parents that she will never marry. Because she is visually presented as a bride at the same time that she rejects marriage, the subliminal message is that her marriage is to her profession, just as a nun's marriage is to Christ or her vocation. Earlier this same evening, Nightingale has yearned to be like Queen Victoria—to be allowed to do a man's work and have a man's point of view. In this scene, she is seated on a chair that is ornate enough to be a throne, with what look like highly stylized crosses on each corner of the chair's back. Visually, then, she has attained her wish: she *is* like a queen on her throne.

The very next scene in the film shows Nightingale at the Fliedner Training School for Nurses in Kaiserswerth, Germany. Two scenes later, Nightingale has returned to London, having finished her training as a nurse. Seeking employment, she proudly presents her diploma to Dr. West, the head of the London hospitals. He brushes her off, telling her that her training will not be wasted because he understands that she is contemplating marriage. In the next scene, England enters the Crimean War. Thus, the film shows Nightingale's instantaneous decision to become a nurse followed immediately by her training at Kaiserswerth, then her application to Dr. West followed immediately by the war. Nightingale's call to the Crimea comes soon after.

This extreme condensation cannot begin to convey the incredible endurance and persistence of Nightingale's desire and efforts to become a nurse. For more than a decade she struggled against her family's sense of the inappropriateness of her desires. In reality, she did not earn a diploma from Kaiserswerth. She managed to stay there only three months while her mother and sister were taking the waters at Carlsbad; the regular nursing training program at Kaiserswerth required three years.[13] But Nightingale was far better prepared for the challenges at Scutari than the film shows her to be. She did not have a diploma, but she did have years of experience visiting hospitals in major cities throughout Europe. And before she was called to the Crimea, she had finally prevailed over her family and had become the superintendent of a charitable nursing home in Harley Street. By omitting her many years of struggle, despair, and even occasional suicidal depressions, and by condensing the extended study and preparation she undertook for her career, the film reduces her to an impulsive young woman who, with tears in her eyes, gets her way by stomping her foot and raising her voice in righteous indignation.

By this point in the film, three important attributes of Hollywood's image of Nightingale are clear. First, her decision to become a nurse is like a holy vocation, but it is also impulsive and sentimental. Nursing, then, is presented as a vocation: a young woman's vocation. Second, Nightingale has professional credentials, her diploma from Kaiserswerth. Thus, nursing is shown as a profession certified by the establishment. The nurse's skills are academic or learned, as well as innate in women. Third, the opposition to her career choice arises from the attitude that a more appropriate role for her is wife and mother. Nursing is an occupation that is similar to wife-and-motherhood, but it requires the sacrifice of that possibility.

Like time, characters are also condensed in the film. For example, Strachey writes of two young men: an early, unnamed suitor (identified by others as Richard Monckton Milnes) to whom Nightingale found herself much attracted; and later, an aristocratic young gentleman who came to Scutari with the romantic notion of serving Nightingale, his idealized heroine. The reception he received from Nightingale was not at all what he had envisioned. She first refused to see him, then consented, but took notes of their conversation and insisted that he sign them at the end of it. The gentleman, according to Strachey, returned to England by the next ship.[14]

In the film, both these young gentlemen are combined in the character Charles Cooper. He is presented as Nightingale's early suitor, whose hand she refuses in order to go about her vocation of nursing. He shows up later at Scutari, offering her his services in whatever way she finds need of them. Nightingale sees him, but she refuses to talk with him about his offer until he has been on a tour of the hospitals. When he returns, he is suitably chastened and tells her that he could never do the work that she is doing, characterizing it as "woman's work." Instead of returning to England, however, he chooses a man's role, enlisting in the army where he will be of some service. He leaves Scutari, but later reappears in the film as a dying patient in a Crimean hospital. In this Hollywood version, Nightingale enters the hospital just in time to hold him in her arms and hear him call her name before he dies. There is no historical basis for this romantic and sentimental scene. Keeping the suitor Charles in the film for so long emphasizes the romantic temptation that in real life Nightingale had put behind her once and for all by 1850 when she had firmly refused Milnes's offers of marriage.

The episode at Scutari also makes explicit in the film the passivity and femininity of Nightingale's career. Charles, in stereotypical contrast, runs away to a life of action, like other jilted movie heroes. Their deathbed reunion, however, works against the stereotype; Florence displays no tearful reconsideration of the rejected suitor, but the compassion of the nurse for a dying soldier.

The romantic theme is again emphasized by a second, similar combining of two characters in one. The first stories of the need for nurses at

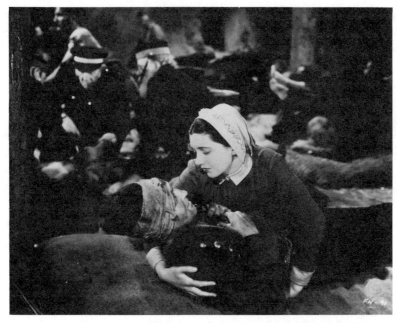

FIGURE 10-2. Kay Francis as Florence Nightingale with a wounded soldier at Scutari. *The White Angel.* Copyright © 1963 Warner Bros. Pictures, Inc. Renewed 1963 United Artists Associated, Inc. Photo courtesy Academy of Motion Picture Arts and Sciences. Reproduced with permission of Turner Entertainment Co.

Scutari were those filed in October 1854 by William Howard Russell, a special correspondent to the London *Times*. The *Times* fund later put at Nightingale's disposal was controlled by a Mr. MacDonald of the *Times*. In the film these two men are fused into one character, a Mr. Fuller, who is both the early correspondent and also the man later in charge of the *Times* fund. Mr. Fuller faithfully does Nightingale's bidding at Scutari and also goes with her to the front lines. After the war, when they have returned to England, he tries to tell her of his feelings for her. She chooses not to understand him, and another movie stereotype is rejected. Faithful service is no more successful in capturing Florence Nightingale than was Charles's dashing gesture.

There are visual reinforcements of this romantic image of Nightingale. The most striking (Fig. 10-2) shows her holding a wounded soldier. She is not engaged in any nursing tasks here. Rather, she holds the soldier tenderly—more as a lover than as a nurse. Her right arm is all the way around his shoulders, her left arm is around his waist, and she looks as if she is about to kiss him. This is the most pronounced visual image in the film of her as a seductive woman, but the men romantically attracted to her reinforce this image.

A third and more subtle combining of characters modifies the romantic motif. Although not mentioned by Strachey, Tommy, the young drummer boy included in the film, is based on a historical character.[15] He was brought wounded into the hospital at Scutari and was nursed by Nightingale. After he recovered, he became her servant and companion, accompanying her everywhere. The film also presents Tommy as one of the patients treated by Nightingale in a famous episode that Cook reports. At Scutari, the doctors used a triage system in deciding which patients to treat. One evening five soldiers were set aside as hopeless. The doctors were too overworked to spend any time on them. Nightingale took over their care throughout the night, and by morning they were sufficiently improved for the surgeons to treat them.[16] The young drummer boy was not one of them. Yet the film's screenwriter makes Tommy the most important of four such patients abandoned by the doctors. Nightingale saves him and the others, and Tommy lives to tell the tale in other parts of the film.

An attractive little boy in the film, Tommy is used to counterbalance Charles Cooper and Mr. Fuller. At one point, he brings Nightingale flowers and asks her if she will marry him when the war is over. She tells him that if she decides to settle down, she will marry him. He thanks her and leaves. By sentimentally presenting the little boy's desire for a romantic relationship with his idealized heroine, the film again emphasizes Nightingale as an attractive young woman. That he is a child, however, lends her the wholesomeness of motherhood.

Events as well as time and characters are condensed and simplified by the movie. Even the film's presentation of a famous legend about Nightingale's opposition to army bureaucracy does not do her justice. In the film, Nightingale seizes by force a consignment of shirts from the government store at Scutari. The factual story given by Cook and Strachey is that in February 1855 the government had sent out 27,000 shirts at Nightingale's request. The shirts were already landed when the medical officers at Balaclava sent a requisition for shirts for the wounded. Nightingale requested them from the purveyor, but the purveyor would not unpack them until after the government's board of survey approved their release. The board of survey did not meet for another three weeks. Meanwhile, the wounded went without shirts. Cook reports an unconfirmed story that Nightingale later ordered a government consignment forcibly opened.

Strachey recounts this story as fact; Cook contents himself with saying that he thinks Nightingale was capable of it.[17]

In the film, this episode of the shirts is slightly altered. Sister Columbo comes to Nightingale and tells her that five hundred shirts are needed for the latest batch of wounded who have come into the hospital. Nightingale tells Sister Columbo to give her the order and follow her. They arrive at the hospital store at seven in the evening and are told by the clerk that the store closes at seven. Nightingale commands him to give her the shirts. He refuses, invoking army regulations. Nightingale then leads her nurses as they break into the store by force and take the shirts they need. Presented this way, the incident is simplified so that it is a question of being one minute too late at the store. Only the clerk's simple-minded adherence to orders stands in the way of the comfort of five hundred wounded soldiers. In reality, the purveyor's simple-minded adherence to orders—not unpacking the shirts until the board of survey met and approved their release—was just the most visible symptom of an overextended imperial government's bureaucratic breakdown. The government's Byzantine bureaucracy led to many such flagrant abuses. The film reduces this bureaucratic maze into the obstinancy of one clerk and prevents the viewer from getting any idea of the formidable organizational obstacles Nightingale really faced. In the film's presentation of her revolt against the clerk, Nightingale is an attractive, sympathetic, and feisty girl-next-door who opposes stupidity by force.

In another condensation of events, the film combines into one trip episodes from Nightingale's three trips to the Crimea. Three incidents are highlighted in the film: first, the medical hierarchy's attempt to starve Nightingale and her nurses by denying them rations; second, Nightingale's vigil in the snow to gain access to one of the Crimean hospitals; and third, Nightingale's bout with cholera. In reality, Nightingale's bout with Crimean fever *did* occur during her first trip to the Crimea, in May of 1855, but the attempt to starve her and her nurses took place on her third trip to the Crimea, in March of 1856. The reports from Alexis Soyer of her standing for hours in the snow while she gave her instructions for the Castle Hospital are probably from her second trip to the Crimea, in October and November of 1855.[18] Fact is the more remarkable: that having been so weakened by Crimean fever, Nightingale would return, not once but twice, to the Crimean front to endure further hardship. The film does not convey her perseverance in this regard.

The incident in which Nightingale and her companions are denied rations is given in the film without any explanation as to how she dealt with

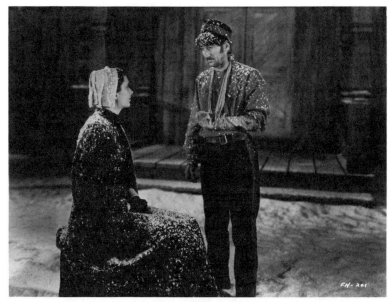

FIGURE 10-3. Kay Francis as Florence Nightingale, with patient, outside the hospital at Balaclava. *The White Angel.* Copyright © 1936 Warner Bros. Pictures, Inc. Renewed 1963 United Artists Associated, Inc. Photo courtesy International Museum of Photography at George Eastman House Still Collection. Reproduced with permission of Turner Entertainment Co.

the situation. In reality, Nightingale had been resourceful enough to bring sufficient rations with her to feed herself and her staff until the dispute could be resolved. In the film, she first appeals to her friend Dr. Scott, who says that he will be court martialed if he helps her. She answers that she can fight for herself, but the scene fades out before any indication is given of how she will do so.

The scene fades to one of her nurses returning from the hospital, saying they have been banned from entering by orders from the diabolical Dr. Hunt, the army's chief medical officer. Nonetheless, Nightingale asks her nurses to follow her to the hospital, as they followed her in the seizing of shirts from the company store. They refuse because they have heard about cholera cases in the hospital and are frightened. Undaunted, Nightingale goes alone to confront the sentry, who will not allow her to enter the hospital. Then she stands in front of the hospital in the falling snow, in full view of the patients, and insists she will stay there until she is permitted to enter. The patients, many of whom recognize her from Scutari, send her a stool to sit on (Fig. 10-3); an officer brings her a cup of tea from the

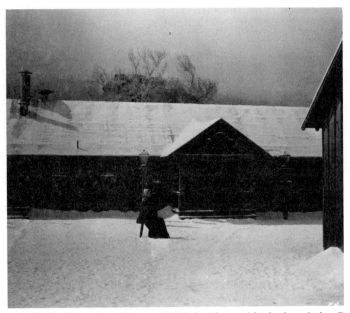

FIGURE 10-4. Kay Francis as Florence Nightingale outside the hospital at Bala-clava. *The White Angel.* Copyright © 1936 Warner Bros. Pictures, Inc. Renewed 1963 United Artists Associated, Inc. Photo courtesy International Museum of Photography at George Eastman House Still Collection. Reproduced with per-mission of Turner Entertainment Co.

officer's mess; and the young drummer boy Tommy gives her his coat and tries to bribe the sentry to let her in. All to no avail. Nightingale sits there in the falling snow (Fig. 10-4) as the patients discuss how long it will take her to freeze to death. The drummer boy asks to see Lord Raglan, the commander-in-chief of the army. When Tommy tells him what's happen-ing, Lord Raglan comes back with Tommy and escorts Nightingale into the hospital.

Other than Soyer's report of Nightingale's standing in the snow for hours giving instructions at the Castle Hospital, the only account in Cook's biography of any such incident comes from one of Nightingale's later letters, April 22, 1869, to a discontented nurse. She recounts among her trials that of having to stand in the snow in front of a hospital to which she had been denied entrance despite the commander-in-chief's orders that she be allowed there.[19] Nightingale was well educated enough to have been familiar with the story of Henry IV of Germany, who, at Canossa in January of 1077, stood barefoot in the snow for three days until he evoked

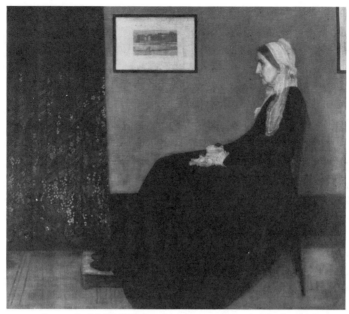

FIGURE 10-5. James A. McNeill Whistler. *Arrangement in Black and Gray: The Artist's Mother*, ca. 1871. Musée d'Orsay. Cliché des Musées Nationaux. Reproduced with permission of Service photographique de la Réunion des musées nationaux.

so much popular sympathy that Pope Gregory VII had to repeal his excommunication order. An apparent humiliation for Henry IV, the incident was really a political triumph for him, removing all obstacles to his rule. Four years later, Henry IV installed his own Pope, Clement III, and Gregory VII had to withdraw into exile in semicaptivity. Likewise, in the film Nightingale turns an apparent humiliation into a brilliant triumph. And in reality, Nightingale's eventual political victories over her opponents were almost as impressive as Henry IV's.

Visually, the most interesting thing about the scene in which Nightingale sits in the snow waiting to gain entrance to the hospital is its evocation of James A. McNeill Whistler's famous painting of his mother (Fig. 10-5). The posture of the two women is very similar, and from a distance Nightingale's headgear appears similar to that of Whistler's mother. Even the basically flat background in the painting is repeated in the scene in the film. Whether the director and producer of the film intentionally set out to call to mind Whistler's painting or not, the scene does so. Since

Whistler's painting of his mother had been exhibited in Chicago in conjunction with the 1933 World's Fair, many people in the United States would have been recently familiar with it, having had the opportunity to see it just three years before this film was released. A picture of the painting was reproduced in the official guidebook to the Fair, which would have given the image in the painting even wider circulation.[20]

The importance of the evocation of Whistler's painting is that it once more identifies mothers with nursing. The painting is widely admired for its masterful presentation of character in art, its capturing of the pathos of the old woman's religious strength and serenity, as well as her calm resignation.[21] The scene in the film does the same for Nightingale. Sitting, as she does, in front of the hospital at Balaclava, Nightingale evokes such sympathy that even the medical hierarchy of the British army has to give way. This is a personal and emotional triumph for the film's heroine. She has won a victory over the evil Dr. Hunt and the impersonal, uncaring bureaucracy by arousing sympathy for her passive persistence in the face of injustice. The mother of nursing is not portrayed as a politically shrewd administrator—which Nightingale actually was—but as a suffering servant who prevails through moral force.

Another interesting aspect suggested by the official title of Whistler's painting, *Arrangement in Black and Gray,* is that *The White Angel,* a black-and-white film, seems in many of its scenes like an arrangement in black and white (and gray). This arrangement is not only visual, but also moral. The film is a morality play between the White Angel of the title and the evil doctors dressed in black, especially Dr. Hunt, who represents the historical Dr. Hall. The title forewarns us of the conflict and its resolution.

There are other visual aspects of the film that are worth noting. In particular, there is the scene in which Nightingale is standing between and slightly above Sister Columbo, her second in command in the film, and Mr. Fuller (Fig. 10-6). The audience of the film is told nothing about Sister Columbo's religious affiliation. Her habit and headdress offer the only information about her other than Nightingale's reference, when she was interviewing the nursing applicants for Scutari, to Sister Columbo as belonging to the Order of St. Vincent. Presumably, then, she is a Sister of Charity. These nursing Sisters took vows, but they were only annual vows, and the Sisters were free at the end of each year to return to the world. The Sisters of Charity distinguished themselves from nuns by taking only these annual vows and refusing to be cloistered.[22] In actuality, the only

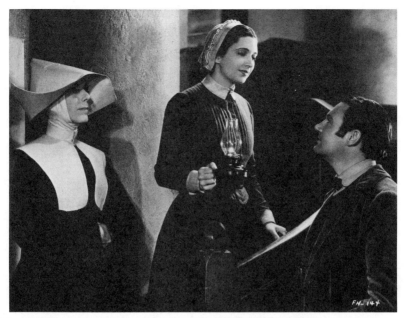

FIGURE 10-6. Eily Malyon as Sister Columbo, Kay Francis as Florence Nightingale, and Ian Hunter as Mr. Fuller, at Scutari. *The White Angel.* Copyright © 1936 Warner Bros. Pictures, Inc. Renewed 1963 United Artists Associated, Inc. Photo courtesy Academy of Motion Picture Arts and Sciences. Reproduced with permission of Turner Entertainment Co.

Sisters of Charity at the Crimea were with the French, not the British, army. The nursing Sisters who accompanied Nightingale were Roman Catholic nuns and Anglican Sisters. The fictional character Sister Columbo is apparently based on the historical Roman Catholic Reverend Mother of Bermondsey, whose help Nightingale found indispensable at Scutari. I cannot explain why the filmmakers changed the nursing order of this character unless it was for aesthetic reasons: to use the visually remarkable headdress of the Sisters of Charity. The film wisely does not explore the intricacies of the various religious orders, nor does it touch on the many problems their conflicts and rivalries presented for Nightingale. As Sister Columbo appears in the film, she stands visually for the traditional Roman Catholic nun.

What makes this scene (Fig. 10-6) so interesting is that Nightingale is poised above and between the two characters who represent the opposed

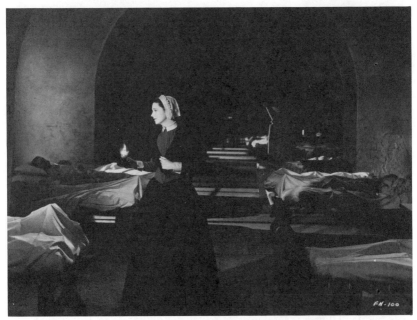

FIGURE 10-7. Kay Francis as Florence Nightingale on her nightly ward rounds at Scutari. *The White Angel*. Copyright © 1936 Warner Bros. Pictures, Inc. Renewed 1963 United Artists Associated, Inc. Photo courtesy Academy of Motion Picture Arts and Sciences. Reproduced with permission of Turner Entertainment Co.

temptations that she is resisting. She chose not to become a religious nun who has taken vows, and she resisted the romantic appeals of men and refused matrimony. Iconographically, this scene is complex. It captures and presents this tension and Nightingale's success in rising above it. Yet, at the same time, it joins the two elements also: Nightingale's profession is both her marriage and her religious vocation.

The scenes in the film that are likely to be remembered longest by the viewers are those that remind them of images they have already seen. These would be the scenes of Nightingale walking through the wards of Scutari at night carrying her lamp (Fig. 10-7), and the image of her standing poised with lamp in hand (Fig. 10-8). These are the most famous images from her story, and they are the ones that have been chosen to represent her and the profession of nursing during most of the ensuing century. While the film shows Nightingale with her lamp on her long walk

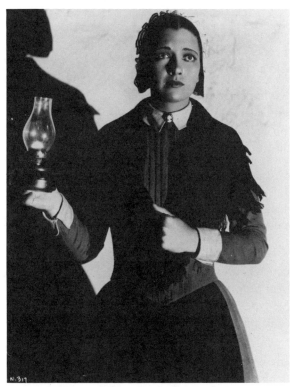

FIGURE 10-8. Kay Francis as Florence Nightingale with her lamp, at Scutari. *The White Angel*. Copyright © 1936 Warner Bros. Pictures, Inc. Renewed 1963 United Artists Associated, Inc. Photo courtesy Academy of Motion Picture Arts and Sciences. Reproduced with permission of Turner Entertainment Co.

through the four miles of corridors at Scutari, several quatrains of Longfellow's poem are recited:

> Whene'er a noble deed is wrought,
> Whene'er is spoken a noble thought,
> Our hearts, in glad surprise,
> To higher levels rise.
> . . . .
> Thus thought I, as by night I read
> Of the great army of the dead,
> The trenches cold and damp,
> The starved and frozen camp—

The wounded from the battle-plain,
In dreary hospitals of pain—
    The cheerless corridors,
    The cold and stony floors.

Lo! in that house of misery,
A lady with a lamp I see
    Pass through the glimmering gloom,
    And flit from room to room.

And slow, as in a dream of bliss,
The speechless sufferer turns to kiss
    Her shadow, as it falls
    Upon the darkening walls.

. . . .

A lady with a lamp shall stand
In the great history of the land,
    A noble type of good,
    Heroic womanhood.[23]

Kay Francis, the 1930s movie star, was in some ways well chosen to represent Nightingale—in other ways, not. Tall and elegant, Francis specialized in Society Maiden movies.[24] Thus, she was able to represent the elegant regal bearing and the graceful walk for which Nightingale was so famous. Francis's beauty, however, was too delicate and soft—made even more so by the occasional soft focus on her face that the filmmakers used—to portray Nightingale's sharpness of features, tongue, and wit. Francis was more like a swan, rather than an eagle, as Strachey characterizes Nightingale.[25] One would expect that qualities associated with Francis in her other films of the times would be carried into her characterization of Nightingale. She was known for her roles as women of wealth and leisure, who succumb to the charms of other men because their husbands are too busy to pay them attention. She made over sixty films of this kind. Her identification with the hint of adultery certainly seems wrong for the character of Nightingale. Perhaps it helps emphasize the contrast with the White Angel who does not succumb.

Warner Brothers, the studio that produced *The White Angel*, was known in the 1930s as the working man's studio. It was also the studio most likely to show working women, but most of its films about working

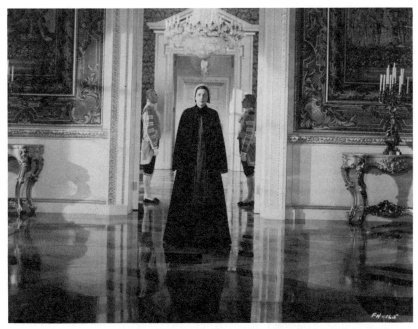

FIGURE 10-9. Kay Francis as Florence Nightingale at the palace of Queen Victoria. *The White Angel*. Copyright © 1936 Warner Bros. Pictures, Inc. Renewed 1963 United Artists Associated, Inc. Photo courtesy International Museum of Photography at George Eastman House Still Collection. Reproduced with permission of Turner Entertainment Co.

women had a sentimental ending that sent the woman out of the work place into the home.[26] With that in mind, it is particularly interesting to consider the ending of *The White Angel*.

In the film, when Nightingale returns to England at the end of the war, she is summoned to an audience with Queen Victoria. Against her mother's wishes, she insists on wearing her nurse's uniform. She rides to the palace in a carriage with Mr. Fuller, who must give her up, and she is encouraged by her old friend Mr. Herbert when she sounds uncharacteristically frightened. The Queen is never shown on the screen. Instead, Nightingale steps forward (Fig. 10-9) and begins to practice her speech while addressing a picture of the Queen. As she speaks, footmen come into the room, take their places, and listen. This ceremonial scene is like a marriage. Nightingale wears her uniform, her special clothing, to the ceremony; Mr. Fuller gives her away; she rehearses for the ceremony; she recites a vow; and in place of a wedding ring, she receives a brooch from the Queen. The film ends with a closeup and then a fadeout on the brooch, which is a cross with Queen Victoria's initials "VR" in the center, topped with diamonds and encircled by the inscription: "Blessed are the merciful."

Nightingale had in fact been sent a brooch just like this by Queen Victoria, but it had come to her by post while she was at Scutari, still recovering from Crimean fever. That this gift is saved to be incorporated into her ceremonial audience with the Queen, makes a very satisfying ending for a film that would have otherwise had to depart from the pattern established in the 1930s. Though Nightingale does not marry in the conventional sense, she does marry her profession and take equivalent vows. At Scutari she had insisted that nurses cannot have a personal life of their own, and she had resolutely sent back to England any nurse who married.

The scene of Nightingale in the palace (Fig. 10-9) is visually complex and very rich, having many components of a Byzantine or Renaissance Madonna. The scene is symmetrical, with balanced paintings and tables on each side. Nightingale is flanked by two servants. Her robes are richly draped, and her headgear is haloed by the white door behind her, pointing upward. The highly polished floor reflects her image, thus accentuating her height, and creates an insubstantial effect, making her seem to float. All these visual elements contribute to the viewer's sense of her as just the opposite of Strachey's demonic character; instead, she is presented here as a transcendent saint.

In the years since 1936 there have been many biographies and studies of Florence Nightingale, including the recent *Florence Nightingale: Reputation and Power* by F. B. Smith, which debunks many of the previously accepted biographical interpretations of her. These later works have nothing to do, however, with the 1936 film. The filmmakers used the best known and most reliable sources available to them, and they cannot be faulted for not knowing what would be written fifty years hence. What is of interest is that even given the impressive research that was done for this film, the alterations that were made all tend toward the same end: making Nightingale a feminine heroine acceptable to the mass audience of her time. In so doing, the filmmakers renewed and enhanced her popular image, but at the cost of portraying her more powerful self.

Most of Nightingale's achievements in the film are sacrificial. The emphasis is continually on what she must give up—marriage, family, a comfortable lifestyle, and so forth. Her accomplishments come through her success in achieving popular sympathy and creating guilt feelings in government officials and occasional army officers. Her passive endurance, shown most dramatically in the scene in the snow in front of the hospital at Balaclava (Fig. 10-4), is one of her major attributes. She is willing to act as a martyr for her cause.

For the thousands of unemployed nurses in the 1930s, this image of self-sacrificing service may have helped give dignity and significance to their hardships. But it is an image that bears only a superficial likeness to the historical Nightingale. The important ingredients of the image owe much to other 1930s Hollywood images of nurses,[27] but they owe most to the powerfully recurring archetypal images of the nurse as mother, seductress, and nun. Although this popular self-sacrificing image of Nightingale is certainly more positive and inspiring than earlier images of nurses, the image has arguably outlived its usefulness to the profession it helped create. Many nurses now reject this image as outmoded nightingalism and consider it harmful to nursing.[28]

The good nurse is not the White Angel; she is more like the real Nightingale—idealistic but also pragmatic, independent, assertive, and resourceful. These are the qualities of Nightingale that should be emphasized as contemporary nursing seeks an image that can inspire young women to become nurses.[29] It is time to reclaim the heritage of the historical Nightingale. Ironically, the spiritual descendants of the real Nightingale are those who have rejected nightingalism.

Notes

1. For a historical illustration of Florence Nightingale with her lamp at Scutari, see Natalie Boymel Kampen's essay in this volume, chap. 1, fig. 1-22.
2. For a discussion of Sairey Gamp, see Leslie A. Fiedler's essay in this volume, chap. 4, pp. 100–112.
3. See "The Lady with the Lamp," *New York Times*, 21 June 1936, sec. 9, p. 4, col. 3–4.
4. Susan Ware, *Holding Their Own: American Women in the 1930s* (Boston: Twayne, 1982), 178.
5. For the announcement of the premiere, see "First Showing of 'The White Angel,'" *American Journal of Nursing* 36 (June 1936): 634; for the stills from *The White Angel*, see *American Journal of Nursing* 36 (May 1936): 574–75.
6. "The Florence Nightingale International Foundation," *American Journal of Nursing* 36 (August 1936): 797.
7. Eleanor W. Mumford, "*The White Angel*," *Public Health Nursing* 28 (August 1936): 540–41.
8. Ibid., 541.

9. See, for example, Frank S. Nugent, "The Screen: A Worshipful Biography of Florence Nightingale Is 'The White Angel,' at the Strand," *New York Times,* 25 June 1936, Amusements section, p. 24, col. 1; and Richard Bertrand Dimmet, *A Title Guide to the Talkies: A Comprehensive Listing of 16,000 Feature-Length Films from October 1927–December 1963* (New York: Scarecrow Press, 1965).

10. Lytton Strachey, *Eminent Victorians* (1918; rpt. New York: Harcourt Brace & World, 1969), 135.

11. Ibid., 136.

12. Sir Edward Cook, *The Life of Florence Nightingale,* 2 vols. in 1 (New York: Macmillan, 1942), 1:13–14.

13. Deborah MacLurg Jensen, *History and Trends of Professional Nursing,* 3d ed. (St. Louis: C. V. Mosby, 1955), 147–48, 126–29.

14. Strachey, 140, 158.

15. Cook, 1:256.

16. Ibid., 1:235.

17. Strachey, 151; Cook, 1: 202–3.

18. Cook, 1:284.

19. Cook, 2:195.

20. *Official Guide: Book of the Fair, 1933* (Chicago: A Century of Progress, 1933), 106.

21. See, for example, Elisabeth Luther Cary, *The Works of James McNeill Whistler* (New York: Moffat, Yard & Company, 1907), 74; and Sadakichi Hartmann, *The Whistler Book: A Monograph of the Life and Position in Art of James McNeill Whistler* (Boston: L. C. Page & Company, 1910), 144–47.

22. For a brief history of the Sisters of Charity, see Jensen, 77–78; for an illustration of their headdress, see M. Patricia Donahue, *Nursing: The Finest Art* (St. Louis: C. V. Mosby, 1985), 221.

23. Henry Wadsworth Longfellow, "Santa Filomena," *Atlantic Monthly* 1 (November 1857): 22–23, lines 1–4, 13–28, 37–40.

24. Marjorie Rosen, *Popcorn Venus* (New York: Avon Books, 1973), 185.

25. Strachey, 141.

26. Molly Haskell, *From Reverence to Rape: The Treatment of Women in the Movies* (Harmondsworth, England, and Baltimore: Penguin Books, 1973), 139.

27. For a discussion of other 1930s films about nurses, see Philip A. Kalisch and Beatrice J. Kalisch, "The Image of the Nurse in Motion Pictures," *American Journal of Nursing* 82 (April 1982): 607.

28. See, for example, Janet Muff's essay in this volume, chap. 9, pp. 197–220.

29. Of interest in this regard is the article by Claire Fagin and Donna Diers, "Nursing as Metaphor," *New England Journal of Medicine* 309 (14 July 1983): 116–17, in which they choose as "metaphor" for themselves Florence Nightingale, because she is "tough, canny, powerful, autonomous, and heroic" (p. 117).

Index

Permissions for Quotations